HEALING MY DIVINE SELF

Opening the Gate
for Life's Purpose

NANCYLITA ALLAN

First published by Busybird Publishing 2021

Copyright © 2021 Nancylita Allan

Print: 978-1-922691-29-3

E-book: 978-1-922691-30-9

Nancylita Allan has asserted her right under the Copyright, Designs and Patents Act 1988 to be identified as the author of this work. The information in this book is based on the author's experiences and opinions. The publisher specifically disclaims responsibility for any adverse consequences, which may result from use of the information contained herein. Permission to use information has been sought by the author. Any breaches will be rectified in further editions of the book.

All rights reserved. No part of this publication may be reproduced, stored in or introduced into a retrieval system, or transmitted in any form, or by any means (electronic, mechanical, photocopying, recording or otherwise) without the prior written permission of the author. Any person who does any unauthorised act in relation to this publication may be liable to criminal prosecution and civil claims for damages. Enquiries should be made through the publisher.

Cover image: Busybird Publishing
Cover design: Busybird Publishing
Layout and typesetting: Busybird Publishing
Editor: Tom O'Connell

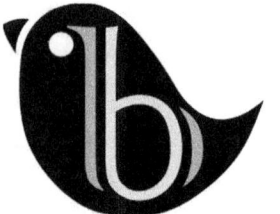

Busybird Publishing
2/118 Para Road
Montmorency
Australia 3094

www.busybird.com.au

DISCLAIMER: Every effort has been made to correctly attribute all quotes within. Any misattributions are unintentional.

About the Author:

Nancylita was born in the Philippines and was the seventh of nine siblings. She migrated to Australia in 1985, seeking to gain a higher education and quality of life. During this time, she earned diplomas in a number of skills and modalities (e.g. aromatherapy, craniosacral therapy, forensic healing, reflexology, remedial massage therapy and Reiki). Nancylita discovered her gift for energy healing by way of her own personal circumstances. In her personal life she reached a point where she required a clearing of negative energy – both physical and emotional – to move forward.

Nowadays she successfully conducts workshops in connection with whole-body and angel healing, as well as other modalities at which she is certified.

Nancylita is married to Norm Allan and resides in Adelaide South Australia. She has one daughter who is married with two children.

Testimonials

'I originally went to see Nancy for a foot reflexology treatment for general health. I mentioned that I was getting nosebleeds *all the time* and Nancy immediately worked towards an appropriate treatment. She performed this treatment and taught me how to do it. I was sceptical at first, but had nothing to lose!

As I got a nosebleed I did what Nancy showed me – and it made the bleeding stop! I continued doing the technique daily for a week or two and the nosebleeds stopped happening altogether! It was easy, unobtrusive and painless!

If you've ever had regular nosebleeds, you know how debilitating it is. Everyone is concerned and makes a fuss, telling you what to do. My doctor thought cauterisation was the only answer! It makes such a difference to be on top of it. I can't thank Nancy enough! I think she is *magic*, really!'

Kyle G.
Glenalta, SA

'I have suffered nose blockages that have led to sleep apnoea. After a session with Nancylita, my blocked left nostril began allowing airflow. For the first time in many years, I felt cold air through my sinuses. It was wonderful. Thank you, Nancylita.'

Lea Q.
Geelong, Victoria

I have been a client of Nancylita Allan's for approximately twelve months. I attend her practice once a month, confident that the right guidance will ensue. I felt trust from my very first session, along with both her wisdom and connection to energies unseen.

Nancylita is an amazing Light Worker.

She is clearly guided by the divine and is a benevolent celestial being who acts as an intermediary between Heaven and Earth.

I leave each session assured and guided on my life's journey, knowing that I am not alone in all realms, physically, emotionally and spiritually.

Nancylita's hands-on healing and angelic guidance is a non-negotiable staple of my life's support network and I will continue to recommend her to my friends and clients alike.'

Denise Dunn
Brighton, South Australia

'Nancy was absolutely amazing when she performed her distant healing over the phone to me. I was in a great deal of pain after the removal of a back molar. She told me to do a breathing routine and I couldn't believe how much it eased the tension. She was fantastic.'

Hannah G.
Adelaide, SA

'Nancy truly is a gifted with healing hands. I have seen Nancylita on various occasions for neck and back pain. When I leave, I feel like I am floating on a cloud.

Thank you, Nancylita.'

Lorraine G.
Adelaide, SA

'I was diagnosed with tongue and throat cancer in August 2012. My surgery was extremely invasive. After a full neck dissection, tongue reconstruction and skin graft I had to have extensive chemotherapy and radiotherapy. I lost the ability to consume normal food and found it difficult to speak. I was in constant pain and was only able to sleep in one-and-a-half hour blocks. I became angry, depressed and anxious. I was glad to be alive but upset that my life had changed so drastically. I had lost my faith and my drive to be happy.

Following my treatment, I was referred to Nancy for some extra support. She developed a holistic treatment plan using reflexology, remedial massage, and craniosacral therapy techniques.

This gave me very quick relief and improved my quality of life.

By utilising spiritual methods, Nancy also helped me regain my sense of self and worth. My saliva was the first thing that I noticed improvements on, followed by improvement to the stiffness and pain in my shoulders and neck. My sleeping patterns improved and I became able to consume small amounts of regular food again. I began to regain strength and movement in my shoulders and arms. I put on weight and my speech and general health improved. I began playing sport again as my energy levels improved. I eventually started back at work after approximately ten months off.

Most of all, I started to feel happy again. I found the value in my life and desired success and happiness. I will never be the same person I was before my surgery, but I have come to be happy and proud to be the person I am now.

Thanks, Nancy.'

Eugene P.
Adelaide, SA

'I was suffering for quite a long time with bursitis in my left shoulder, which meant that I couldn't lift my arm or reach behind me without experiencing excruciating pain. The doctors wanted to give me Cortisone injections, but I was hesitant as these had never helped me in the past.

Doctors didn't want me to have any additional treatment, as they said that it would 'interfere' with their program. Well, their program wasn't working and I was still in too much pain to sleep. Nothing had changed for over six months.

Well, Nancy then went on a course over the weekend to learn a new technique called Muscle Tension Reset, which sounded good! She was fascinated by the whole thing and was dying to try it out on somebody. It looked like that someone would be me…

To be honest, I thought she was joking when she started the treatment, as she just started brushing my shoulder lightly with her fingers and that was it! Well, blow me down, but after ten minutes of this 'treatment' (haha) the pain went away! I promised not to take the Mickey again and it was a good week. After some night time discomfort, pain crept back into the shoulder, so Nancy gave me another session, which took another fifteen minutes.

No lie: I have never had even a twinge of pain in my shoulder since. Not once! That was the end of that story, nearly five years ago! Nancy is simply magic and this was not the only time that she helped me.

I was recently plagued with a stiff neck that would not go away! Oh my god, it was so intrusive! And being here in the UK, autumn in full swing, I couldn't just hop in the car and go crying to Nancy, could I?

So when I mentioned it to her, she asked if I would mind if she tried to help from *there*, while I was *here*! I had nothing to lose, Nance guided me through what I had to do while on the phone. Five minutes later, I was feeling much better and the next morning I couldn't believe it; the pain was completely gone!

What I can say? Magic as ever :)'

Peter G.
United Kingdom

'After surgery to treat my tongue and throat cancer, I visited Nancy to see if she could help my body recuperate. I wanted to be normal and healthy again. The treatment I received from Nancy has improved my body functions, specifically my damaged salivary glands.

My doctor was very pleased with the results and I have since continued treatment with Nancy. I've noticed my negative energy has cleared and my whole being has improved.'

Dennis C.
Adelaide, SA

'I initially sought Nancy's assistance after suffering an anxiety attack in 2011. I have continued to visit and receive regular therapy since.

Nancy's friendly ongoing therapy (to address various minor ailments) has made a significant difference to my lifestyle. Therefore, it is without hesitation that I would recommend Nancy's support and therapy.'

John H.
Adelaide, SA

'Nancy Allan is a very spiritual, gifted person with powerful hands. Her reflexology treatment can help a lot of people. She has helped me and others out in ways I couldn't imagine. I truly believe without Nancy I would be in dire health straits.

Thanks so much Nancy for all you've done for me.'

Dimos K.
Perth, WA

'For many years I have suffered muscle tension in my neck and shoulders. This has caused me back pain and general discomfort.

I have tried various treatments with varying results. Recently I consulted with Nancylita Allan, who I feel is finally giving me some relief and I am able to cope with the pain and discomfort better.

I would have no hesitation in recommending her to anyone suffering similar problems.'

Faye S.
Prospect, SA

'One morning I woke with a very bad headache. I don't know what caused it, but I tried all the natural remedies, like food, water and rest, but they didn't work. I even tried painkillers, but the effects were just temporary.

That night, I visited Nancy and told her what was going on. She applied pressure to my legs, clearing my head and easing the pain! She told me this was simple acupressure, and... I don't really understand what the principle is, but it was great.

I have recommended Nancy to all my friends. Whatever ailment you have, go and see her. I'm sure she will be able to help you out.'

Tony
Blair Athol, SA

'I had my neck treated by Nancy Allan. I could not move it much, as it was stiff and sore. To my amazement, I feel ninety-five percent better now. The best part was I experienced no pain when she did her treatment!

I am now one of her regular customers!'

Dora P.
Adelaide, SA

'My mother referred me to Nancy because she could see something wasn't quite right with me. I felt nauseous a lot of the time and trips to the doctor weren't helping. Mum brought me to Nancy and at first I was nervous and my stomach was unsettled. Nancy talked me through what she does and explained her background and experience. Her explanation, warm manner and the atmosphere of the room calmed me right away. We got started on the reflexology and relaxation techniques. Surprisingly my nausea began to fade and I had the energy of a five-year-old. I felt the negativity and sickness leave my body. It was amazing. I felt refreshed and new.

Nancy has done an absolutely marvellous job. I really look forward to future sessions. I love feeling so young again.'

Alicia H.
Adelaide, SA

'I went to see Nancy as I felt my back beginning to tighten up. I do a lot of manual handling at work and feared I was losing my flexibility, which is essential for safe manual handling. I was also feeling "down" and "negative" generally.

Nancy gave me a long session, massaging my spine and muscles to unknot some points. She then did a reflexology therapy on my feet. I felt better immediately and Nancy gave me some advice on simple meditations and natural foods to stimulate health and wellbeing.

Two weeks later I can say my back has been fine and I have regained my natural flexibility and sense of joy and wellbeing.'

Helen H.
Adelaide, SA

'For over six months I suffered from Bursitis of the right hip. This was always painful and made it difficult for me to sleep. The throbbing pain was constant and, on a scale from one to ten, was a nine.

After Nancy's treatment, the pain was immediately halved! In the days and nights that followed I felt even better. (Oh my god, I even slept and could at last enjoy my bed again!) Now the pain is almost completely gone. I am back in the gym and can walk without discomfort, all after just one treatment!

I am over the moon with these results. Nancy has magic healing hands! I am really impressed with her professionalism, courteousness and trustworthiness.

I have already recommended her to many friends and family. I have also signed up for a regular "service" and joined her meditation class after my first visit.'

Keryn W.
Adelaide, SA

'My personal experience with Aromatherapy massage has been wonderful. I was amazed at how fast it brought relief to the horrible ache in my neck, which I had suffered for many years.

I am a very active athletic woman in my forties with five boys. After years of really pushing myself to the limit, and after many visits to various medical teams trying to find relief, I came across Nancy.

After leaving the clinic that first day I felt something I hadn't felt in a long time: hope. The tenderness and severe ache that interfered with my everyday life was subsiding after a very short time. Nancy also helped relieve my stress during this very challenging time in my life.

My visits to Nancy have become a weekly highlight. I thought I would have to put up with neck pain for the rest of my life, but her techniques, advice and guidance cured them. I have since recommended Nancy to my mother and auntie and their outcome, like mine, has been amazing.

Thank you, Nancy Allan, for sharing your knowledge and professional conduct with us. Also for your sincerity to help others, which, in itself, is a godsend. God bless you always!'

Vessy T.
Parafield Gardens, SA

'Nancy is a highly skilled and gifted reflexology and massage therapist. I've been a client since November 2010 and have always received first-class treatment in a caring and supportive manner.

Nancy has created a very nurturing environment for clients. She always asks me what I feel I need when I arrive. I've received benefit from relaxation massage, aromatherapy, reflexology and other treatments where Nancy has prepared specific products for my healing. She respects me, my knowledge of my body and how I'm feeling. Together we work out the most suitable solution for my health issue at the time.

Even when I don't believe I have any specific thing that needs attention, Nancy can quickly identify blockages in my energy flow and release them. Her exceptional intuition in connecting with me and my body is a very special gift that she willingly shares.

After receiving treatment from Nancy, I found a real improvement in all areas of my body and my mental alertness. Following a car accident, I required treatment and my shoulder, neck and back flexibility improved immensely thanks to Nancy's gentle and targeted treatment program.

I appreciated Nancy's genuine care for me and her interest in helping solve my health challenges. I also appreciate the ongoing learning she undertakes to provide the latest and most suitable treatment options for her clients.

I feel blessed to have Nancy on my wellness team and highly recommend her to everyone who is ready to enjoy improved health and wellness.'

Gabi P.
St Agnes, SA

'I was suffering from what my GP called "Raw Shoulder". I had no relief from the pain or symptoms from any medicine my GP prescribed, so I sought out Nancy to help me. I'm glad I did!

Before the treatment I could hardly use my left arm at all and my neck was frozen. During Nancy's treatment I felt the pain reducing and by the end it was less than half of what it was before! I booked in for a follow-up treatment a week later, but during the next forty-eight hours, I almost completely recovered! I felt so good that I have not had to go back since!

I know who I will be going to for further health advice and treatment. Nancy is an angel!'

Lisa V.
Adelaide, SA

'My name is Rocco. I am eighteen years old and very physically active in a variety of sports. Diet and muscle composition is very important to me. I found Nancy to be very interested and caring in the areas of concern to me. Once addressing these areas, pain and discomfort disappeared. I was extremely happy with Nancy's expertise in muscle tension reset, remedial massage and her customer service approach.'

Rocco C.
Adelaide, SA

'I visited Nancy when I was working as a case manager at a domestic violence service. I was suffering bad headaches and neck and shoulder pains. My blood pressure was also getting high and I had difficulty sleeping. Nancy's massage sessions helped a lot. I then recommended her to some of my workmates and friends and they all gave me inspiring feedback.

I'm now seventy years old and retired. One day I almost fell while weeding in my garden. I suffered terrible pain from my hips down to my knees. I had to hold on to the fence and walls to get inside the house. I panicked and fell on the couch to collect myself and, after an hour, I came to my senses and rang Nancy. She accommodated me and I came to her in my gardening clothes and dirty shoes. I was in too much pain to change. Nancy had to help me take off my shoes, socks, jumper and jeans. She got me to lie on her massage table and applied pressure on my back, hips and foot for less than thirty minutes. Afterwards I was able to get up on my own without pain and put on my clothes, socks and shoes without assistance. I walked out of her clinic as if nothing had happened to me. What magic!'

Joan D.
Blair Athol, SA

Introduction

This book is dedicated to those souls who seek guidance to relieve the doubt or anxiety inhibiting their everyday wellbeing. As a forensic healing practitioner, I offer forensic analysis and spiritual guidance that will clear many blockages to your mind and wellbeing.

I was inspired to write this book after an experience I had parenting my daughter through a near tragic bout of whooping cough. Traditional medical methods seemed to have no effect on her recovery, so I sought guidance from spiritual and divine healing practice to enable recovery to good health. I believe I possess a gift for helping others achieve their goals and hope to share some of what I've learnt with you here.

Disclaimer

Please be advised that the information provided in this book is designed to help with the subjects discussed herein. As stated by the author, these experiences should not be used to replace treatment or for the purpose of self-diagnosing medical conditions. Individuals should make their own independent assessment before acting on any content. It is emphasised that the information provided is not to be taken as legal or medical advice and cannot be reproduced or published by any source without the author's written consent. The content is of a general nature and should not be construed as specific or complete advice.

Note: Names mentioned in this book have been changed for privacy reasons.

Table of Contents

Dedication		1
1	My Story – Journey to Wellness	3
2	The Discovery: Unlocking the Healer	11
3	Chakra Healing – Opening Energetic Centres	17
4	The Angels – Healing Lights	29
5	Energy Blocks – Finding Energy Blocks	41
6	Forensic Energy Healing Revelation of the Healing Secret	47
7	Breaking the Patterns: Universal Attraction	51
8	The Meditation-Mindful Medicine	57
9	Life Purpose – Heal for Purpose	63
10	Bonuses: Divine Self Healing Tips	67
11	Abundance/Finances the Unlimited Source	75
12	The Next Generation	81
Acknowledgement		87
Sources		89

Dedication

I would like to dedicate this book to my loving daughter Carla, who was instrumental in helping me discover my gift as a healer; to my mother, for guiding and supporting her children with wisdom and compassion so that they could best serve humanity; to my siblings, for sharing fun childhood memories with me; to my nephews and nieces for keeping me young at heart; to Emily Jean Waye, my mother-in-law, for her untiring support in our time of need; and to all my clients, casual or regular, for trusting me to be part of their health program and for giving me a broad range of experiences that have helped me on my healing journey.

I would also like to dedicate this to Michelle Mayor for clearing my energy field when I was unable to do so myself, and for further dissipating the negative energy that had become attached to me after a client's treatment. I also give thanks to my angel course teacher Darren Linton, for teaching me how to connect with angels and all-loving spirits, for my miraculous opportunity to meet Jesus and for my out-of-body experiences.

Finally I'd like to thank my spiritual mentors all over the world for guiding me and showing me how to eliminate my limited beliefs. To Marisa Russo, my forensic energy healing teacher, thank you for being an inspiration to women living in darkness. Your course has helped me open up the gates of opportunity, assist more people who are willing to relieve themselves from negative beliefs and, most of all, empower women to see and recognise their full potential.

One

MY STORY – JOURNEY TO WELLNESS

'Imagination is your greatest creative tool.'
– Bob Proctor

When I was five years old, I used to take flowers to the chapel near our house. I inherited this habit from growing up in a Catholic family. My mother maintained a strong devotion to all saints, angels and God, so mass on Sundays was a compulsory occasion for us kids. Other villagers also had to attend this devotion, where children behave differently inside the chapel. Everyone would kneel quietly while communicating with God and, while doing so, I made a request to God. I asked Him to allow me to go abroad when I grew up to seek suitable employment. This way I could assist my family out of the ever-present poverty that existed in the Philippines. Even then it was a common practice for Filipinos to seek employment to improve their life situation. My little mind's plan was to go to Saudi Arabia, as I didn't know of other places to get a job at five years of age. It was just a dream I had before I even started school. Why did I think that way? Maybe it was my adventurous mind, which never runs out of ideas.

When I commenced primary school I always wondered what I would do when I grew up. I always wanted to have a big house as I did not have a room to myself. It was normal to share with siblings, but it would have been nice to have my own room, like the ones I saw in the comics and magazines that were passed around the neighbourhood. Many years later my cousins and I got together at one of our uncle's houses to do some corn kernelling work. While doing so, we talked about our future and what direction we were headed in.

This topic broke down the monotony of corn kernelling. When it was time for bed the five of us slept together on the lounge floor next to a huge pile of corn kernels. Bedtime provided us with giggling and joking and general chatter before we drifted off to sleep, exhausted from our work. At eleven and twelve years of age, it was a fun time full of beautiful childhood memories. When it was time to go to college we went to different institutions. Most of us lost contact and only saw each other once a year, usually around Thanksgiving Day. Our interests varied then, so there was no more corn kernelling. Situations started to improve on my parents' small farm, enabling harvesting and kernelling machines to gradually takeover the jobs we were once called upon to do. In hindsight our parents designed these jobs to keep us out of trouble and mischief.

As I was getting older my vision to go abroad was getting stronger and clearer in my heart. I knew I would not be staying in the Philippines forever. When I finished college I had an urge to go to Manila to find a job as my two brothers were already living there – the youngest still finishing college and the eldest in the army. The divine direction I requested when only a child came to fruition and led me to Australia, not Saudi Arabia, and thankfully so! The opportunity presented itself when I was employed in one of Manila's international hotels. By chance I met my daughter's father, eventually marrying and settling down in this wonderful country, Australia.

Prior to moving to Australia and marrying I was enrolled in an agricultural degree at college. However, I soon realised this was not my full ambition or direction. I describe my time prior to coming to Australia as fun, although it was also a struggle to maintain my everyday routines. This provided me with experiences and guidance and has contributed to the gratitude I feel with my present life situation and life's purpose. This will be elaborated on as I continue; however, let me digress and go back to before I went to Manila to seek a possible better existence, as this situation contributed to the present acknowledgement and pursuit of my life's purpose. I became aware that my mother was suffering from a grave and possibly life-threatening illness. She had never disclosed this to us so suffered and endured this affliction in silence.

Before I went to Manila we were already aware of our mother's condition, but we didn't have the money to get an appropriate medical diagnosis. Because we lived on a farm in a village-type existence, my mother's illness was common knowledge. People still got on with their lives, though, and my mother was good at disguising her plight and dissuading others from giving sympathy. Most people believed everything was okay with her, and life carried on. One time I came upon my parents arguing when I arrived home from school. Ordinarily my mother possessed a calm conversational voice, but this time she was engaged in fierce debate with my father. She was at pains to make a point to my father. Her voice was elevated but as soon as she saw me, she reverted to her normal placid manner. When I asked what the argument was about she impressed upon me that everything was fine, that they were just discussing matters that needed to be attended to around the farm.

When she asked my father nicely to agree to her requests, my father followed her order with a look of disgust. Hiding their arguments was a practice my mother adopted. It may have emanated from the Spanish background on my mother's family side. Disagreements of this kind were rare in our family. In fact, most of the other villagers thought we were made in heaven. As children we sometimes upset each other just being kids and most of the resolutions came from our elders, who encouraged us to give in.

Giving in didn't always come easy, though, and if we could not settle the misunderstanding ourselves punishment would follow. Pushing these emotions down without proper resolutions created sadness and anger inside our bodies, but we learned to suppress our anger and feelings of sadness. In my opinion, adopting this practice of suppressing emotions can upset the balance of homeostasis. If held, it can affect your liver and lungs in the long term. I believe my mother's illness manifested itself because of the long-term negative emotions she held within. This made the whole family feel helpless. We were unaware of how severely this type of illness can affect the heart. I am sure it was just a practice the family had adopted, which had been handed down for generations. My mother was a known pacifist and had love for everyone before herself. She was very religious and spiritual, teaching us to love God above all things. I, being the seventh of nine children, often wondered how she managed to bond with each of us, and left us meaningful experiences and wisdom in our younger years.

My mother had the wonderful ability to display her care and affection to each of us without favouritism. However, tragedy befell us when mother gave birth at a very late age while she was possibly menopausal and against all medical odds. The family rejoiced in this birth and the newest addition seemed to be doing well. However, after two weeks he passed away. The cause of death was attributed to liver failure. It caused a jaundiced condition whereby his skin yellowed and the whites of his eyes arose from the excess pigment bilirubin typically caused by obstruction of the bile duct. Well, my curiosity got me to do further research into this disease. I was at this time studying for an agriculture qualification, which had nothing to do with my curiosity about why a healthy baby suddenly died. I know now that if today's medical facilities and knowledge were available then the baby would have survived.

My brothers and sisters were leaving home before me, one at a time, including those who got married. I watched my mother shed tears over and over every time they left after the holidays and I felt her happiness every time they came home on holidays. She missed them deeply and, when I asked her why she was so emotional, her response was a deep silence. Her love, devotion and wise counsel throughout our lives were impressed upon us all. Of course it is only as I matured and gained life experience that these guidelines and memories from my mother became my inspiration.

As my parents got older their bond weakened and they became more distant. This will be expounded upon in later writings. My mother let us follow our dreams, as there would not be many opportunities for us if we remained around the farm. She guided us to follow the path of God and mothered us through her actions, with few spoken words. However, when she spoke she was full of loving words which were heard and felt. Every syllable was imprinted in our hearts. She went to church on our birthdays and celebrated alone, while we had a real party somewhere else. Her dedication to each and everyone of us was unsurpassed.

She even remembered each of our favourite dishes. When I was in college my mother wished for me to study agriculture. Her intention was for me to manage our farm in a new age after the land's organic content depleted. Rice now had to be grown with the aid of fertilisers. In accordance with my mother's wishes I attended San Miguel Agricultural College, which was south from where we were. It was a cheap college in which students could self-support through rice planting. Additionally, it had given me the opportunity to play with the earth and learn the modern methods of agriculture (in particular, managing a real farm by designing, landscaping and producing rice and vegetables on a quarter acre of land). The Philippine government allowed us to work the land like it was our own until we finished the course.

It wasn't easy and only a few girls completed the term. It was designed so that we would learn to be self-supportive. However, my older siblings helped me as much as they could so it was a little easier for me than for some of the other students. We learned to negotiate to sell our produce before we harvested and got higher grades in agri-business if we sold three quarters of the produce prior to harvesting time, just like real farmers. It was fun but tiring. Most students fell asleep during our classes. On school breaks I visited home and indulged in my favourite mud crabs that my mother fattened up on rice husks. She didn't have an aquarium like most traditional restaurant owners. The idea was brilliant as mud crabs can live in a partial dry area, buried in the rice husks for months. We all loved seafood, so mother organised for local fishermen to save her the best when our homecoming drew closer. My mother was getting thinner as the years went by, although none of us took much notice as she appeared energetic and fit and would run around getting the best food in the market while we were still in bed. Mother was totally absorbed in pleasing us when we were home and our presence seemed to energise her. However, she never complained or revealed her heart and lung disease to us. She suffered silently. I remember most vividly my older brother and I (before he was accepted into the army) did not come home one night on separate occasions. Our mother searched everywhere in the village houses, walking miles using only a kerosene lamp as her light.

We were well-behaved children because of our upbringing and mother's guidance. We learned to please everyone and ensured we were modest and that we chose the right words in conversation. My mother's will and determination for us to succeed was most evident when extended family members asked us to assist them with harvesting and associated house chores. She was very compassionate and the most respected woman in the whole village. This very calm placid woman managed to conquer the hearts of many and possessed the strongest appearance in the whole community. She had loving concern for everyone in the village and was well known for her caring nature and habit of putting others first.

As I remember all this, tears run down my face. I wish she could still be here to share life with me and my beautiful family, enjoying a rewarding life that she never experienced. Even though I feel she is with me in spirit, the lessons she taught me and the attributes I have inherited from my mother, like her love of life, have encouraged me to find the true meaning of love. Her big heart provided light not only for her children but to all the lives she connected with, even as she battled her own darkness.

My catholic practice has waned so much and I no longer attend church as often as I was brought up to do. I consider myself a very spiritual person, but not a religious one. The martyr concept – which is how my mother chose to walk her life – was never intentional, but it was my guide to finding the truth about how to connect with God and understand the real meaning of His love. As a mother myself, I now fully understand her behaviour, her concern for her children, and how this limited insight tipped out her equilibrium. 'The things we do for love,' they say, forgetting that we also have needs.

The seriousness of my healing journey started when my daughter was only a toddler. She went very suddenly from a very healthy, happy baby who was adored by everyone to a sick baby. Sadly, medical doctors couldn't help. All they could do was write prescriptions. There was no doubt our general practitioner was doing his best to help but he could only help so much. My husband and I took turns minding her as we could not continue leaving a sick baby to babysitters and my mother-in-law. Although my beautiful mother-in-law spent so much time helping, I often took sick leave from work to spend time with my daughter. She got used to this and, as she got older, she often told me to take a sickie to spend time with her.

My daughter's illness was just an assortment of infections. Some parents would say it wasn't too serious, as they say children go through illnesses to build up their immune systems, which could be true. However, my daughter's defence mechanisms were not responding to medications and, upon watching her suffer through a whooping cough, poor appetite and a fever that persisted despite medication, I was afraid her condition could lead to more serious complications. I feared she would become a medical trial guinea pig to find a cure for what were supposed to be familiar illnesses.

One day on the way to get more antibiotics, I prayed for guidance from Heaven and asked for help from the divine source. It was my last resort. My mother once told me to pray and ask for spiritual intervention in time of desperation.

We passed a book sale just before heading to the chemist. We stopped to have a browse and I saw this foot reflexology book. My heart pounded as I held it. A strange power flashed over me. I opened it at random. Coincidentally the page I opened to described problems similar to my daughter's. A strong gut feeling told me to buy this book, so no mucking around; the decision was made. I was excited. I then found another surprise when I got to the counter to pay. The book was heavily discounted. In my excitement, I went home, forgetting to buy the medication.

When we got home I could hardly wait to start reading. I followed the techniques and applied them on my daughter's foot. While concentrating, I glanced at my daughter's face. She seemed to be enjoying the foot massage, even though the technique was not yet natural to me. I concentrated on the reflex point corresponding to the lung organ for her unheard-of long-term cough. It was located on the footpad below the toes. According to the book, this would alleviate the condition. As I continued, I noticed my daughter was responding to the treatment. Her pale skin started to changed, her circulation improved and her coughing settled. Within less than a day, she'd shown slight improvement. She even asked for food – a sign that her appetite was returning. I never left her side and encouraged her to eat more. My mother used to do the same, giving us full attention when we were not well. She would always tell us to ask for anything we craved and she would make sure she fulfilled our body's demand as this would support and speed up the healing process.

Three days passed and my daughter got better without the prescribed medicines. From that moment my life changed. I became humbler and more appreciative of life and all that we had. When I see children coughing, I straight away offer to touch their feet. While attending my daughter's birthday party, my girlfriend's daughter began coughing non-stop. I came out with a bucket of warm water with a few drops of peppermint oil and asked the child to soak her feet to soften them. I then started performing foot reflexology and the cough switched off in just a few minutes. She'd had it for weeks.

My daughter's episode in 1992 helped me realise my calling. It was a hint from above which I hadn't paid attention to in my younger days. I remember when my mother and I went to visit one of her aunties. We walked a few kilometres and, as I was just a little girl, my mum held my hand so I would keep up with her pace. Her hand started to warm up as soon as she touched me and soon turned hot. She thought I was sick. This happened many times. My hands would feel very hot and only my mother would notice. When we'd get home she'd tell my father I was unwell and that I was not allowed out to play with my siblings and neighbours because I was coming down with a cold. Because of this, I associated this feeling of heat emitting from my hands with a feeling of unfairness. Why did I have to be kept inside the house while everyone else enjoyed themselves outdoors? I used to fight with my mum about this because I felt perfectly fine. My dad would feel my head and it was okay, but my mother would worry what might happen if I was exposed to the weather outside. Typical mother, she was.

As I spent more time practising it, my interest in performing reflexology became a natural talent. People recognised my ability and came to me for treatment. At that time, I mostly treated coughs when prescribed medicine was not effective.

On one occasion, Cherie brought her four-year-old daughter to our place for a foot reflexology treatment. We were living in the South Australian hills at the time. Her daughter had a persistent cough that would not subside. The little girl felt unwell and this was slowly affecting the balance of her family. While performing the treatment, her daughter felt very relaxed and fell asleep on my reclining chair. She was silent, with no more coughing. We left her to sleep after the treatment and, while waiting, Cherie asked if reflexology could help her get pregnant for a second time. She had already tried many avenues with no success. This was something I did not expect but, I thought, why not? I did her treatment right at that moment while sitting on another reclining chair waiting for her daughter to wake up. It became a normal routine for me to help everyone. I felt it was my duty as I was so grateful to have found a way to help my daughter and maintaining her health. The people I have treated insisted on paying for my work. I accepted these blessings and signs of gratitude, as they call it. Word of mouth quickly spread and I became more popular. I decided I had better get a proper certification before I got in trouble from other therapists or natural therapy associations.

I started studying casually on the weekend. I completed workshops until I found the proper school to grant me certification. There, at the Natural Health Academy (NHA) in South Australia, I obtained my first diploma in Reflexology. Reflexology became my passion. Even today it is still my favourite modality. I really enjoy it and recommend it to all my clients for maintaining high immunity levels.

The art of healing encouraged me to expand and learn different modalities. This led me to further learning and the obtainment of more diplomas in aromatherapy, craniosacral therapy, remedial massage therapy, Reiki and, finally, forensic energy healing, which I found the most powerful healing modality.

Two

THE DISCOVERY – UNLOCKING THE HEALER

'Scars have the strange power to remind us that our past is real.'
– Cormac McCarthy, All the Pretty Horses

Healers are interconnected and are no different to anyone else who needs healing. I have seen various practitioners to deal with my blockages and did not realise how seriously they affected my life. My whole being was healed and layers of negative life patterns, which were preventing me from living the life of my dreams, were released.

My connection with angels, my past healing experience and the divine guidance I received from my precious daughter's health, made me realise I have the gift of warm hands. This is what my daughter experienced when I touched her. She often complimented me on how nice it was to be touched with warm hands whenever she had a foot massage. When she got better I noticed my hands weren't as warm anymore. I had this realisation while reflecting back on my younger days. Why and how did I possess warm hands? My mother discovered this when I was young. She believed that hot or warm hands indicated I was coming down with a fever or illness. Ironically, back then my warm touch indicated my mother was suffering from tuberculosis and a heart condition, things that eventually brought about her premature death. Of course at that age I did not know the significance of warm hands, but this was another discovery that enabled me to seek divine explanation.

After more than ten years experience as a healer I am also learning to recognise negative life patterns that exist in my relationships, particularly after divorcing my daughter's father. Ongoing relationships that I had attracted were ending in a similar fashion. Why was this? At that time the main thing I noticed was the negativity after their wooing succeeded. Most of my relationships lasted five to six years, and what were the reasons for this hiatus? Upon analysis it was purely that I did not know what I was searching for – not only in relationships but in life. Once I had recognised and addressed this fact life entered into a different, more enjoyable phase. You have to see the dirt to clean it. Physical discomfort started to dissipate. Through the modality of forensic healing I have released layers of negative energies that I never knew existed and, at the same time, discovered my life purpose. The guidance of Jesus and the angels became clear to me; it is our choice and responsibility to create the lives we want to live. When I studied the Angel course taught by Darren Linton, my deep meditation experiences involved visiting the angelic realm and having a party with all my favourite angels and archangels. Each of them had different tasks for me when I called upon them. Every time I need guidance in a situation, a Divine Mercy image comes into mind.

The healer Archangel Raphael guides me to choose the modality most suited for my client's particular discomfort. This makes my healing work faster, easier and more effective. The excitement I feel when meeting new clients is always weird and spooky. This is also how a friend described it as I helped him through a distant healing. His affliction, a fragile Achilles tendon, gave the sensation of a loss of strength and pain. In communication, his discomfort was relieved by controlled breathing and healing energy transported via his mobile phone connection. Well, that incident had given me the opportunity to practise my distant healing using Reiki energy healing. I guided him to breathe deeper with me at the same time, directing my energy to his pain. After five minutes he told me that he was better and could walk around the kitchen.

Because I am guided to help my clients heal, my work is never boring. I always look forward to treating clients, using myself as a conduit in the healing process. I am also fuelled by the fresh energy coming through me from the Divine source as I perform the healing. In my early days of healing using reflexology, one of my friends bought a voucher for her friend, Donna, who was forty-two years of age and wanting a simple relaxing massage. Having just finished an aromatherapy course, I felt this was a chance to practise my massage techniques. As per my usual procedure, I asked her a few questions before mixing the oils. I asked if she was pregnant or thinking of getting pregnant. Aroma therapists are required to ask this before undergoing treatment for safety reasons. She answered that at her age she needed to give up wanting to have children after trying unsuccessfully for many years. I suggested she try reflexology after her full-body massage. She agreed and I was then guided to concentrate on her ovarian and uterine points.

Six months later my girlfriend, who had bought Donna a voucher, came to see me for a treatment. She told me the good news: Donna was pregnant with a baby boy! Both Donna and her husband were very happy. She no longer believed she would ever get pregnant. Life is full of surprises. I felt proud and confident in my healing gift.

Not long after I was visited by Julia, who lived and worked across the road from my clinic. Julia had been married for more than five years and seriously wanted to have a child. She and her husband had already visited a few natural therapists and had been told that babies come in their own time. Julia booked in to discuss her situation with me. She was only on her mid-twenties, but wanted to have a family before she turned thirty. We organised ongoing regular treatment. She preferred foot reflexology as it gave her the total relaxation she needed after her tiring work as an accountant.

When she came for her fourth monthly session, she had some surprising news: she was pregnant. She said it was safe to tell me now that she was over three months along and she was surrounded by loving spirits, including my three brothers from the other side.

I have so much fun on my healing journey. When following guidance it is so much easier to deal everyone's discomforts, which could be distorting relationships. This leads me to the next client story.

Jean, a divorced mother of two, came to see me. She felt sad because her eldest daughter had grown distant ever since Jean had found a new partner. They were both suffering from the situation. I was guided to clear her negative emotions and heal her energy field using Reiki. I then followed this with foot reflexology to support her internal organs. The treatment made her feel relaxed and at peace. She organised for her daughter Mely to have a session two days after. When I saw Mely I immediately noticed that she had a full load of emotions – notably anger. With my judgemental side, I sensed she had a controlling attitude. I asked if she'd come to see me for herself or for her mother. She said it was for herself, which allowed us to move on and start the healing process. I wanted to clear all of her negative emotions, which are not beneficial to a mother-daughter relationship. I used craniosacral therapy as a guide and calmed her by performing a transverse plane. It did not take long for her to become relaxed.

I needed her to be in this state so that her body would follow and allow healing to occur. While she was in her deepest state of relaxation, I started asking which negative emotions she was experiencing from my lists. I told her to answer 'no' if she did not feel that emotion and 'yes' if it was affecting her. I also told her to let go of the negative emotions as we identified them.

After the session Mely was calmer and more relaxed. She booked another session for the following week. When I next saw her she was a lot happier. This family was the first I helped to clear emotional distortion. The way the spirits help is so miraculous. I have learned to trust and follow their guidance. I also physically experience the transformation, treating aches and pains as I follow along with the guides. Every session is just divine and leaves me feeling calm and content when it finishes. During Mely's second session I did transverse planes again. I closed my eyes to deepen my concentration and communicated with the divine source. I asked for assistance from the angels, and for the best and highest guides. They mostly come in groups and I enjoy their company, including my late family.

Mely did some deep breathing to relax. Following my instructions, she breathed through her nose to activate her nitric oxide hormones. This helped her body relax, so it could repair and rejuvenate the damage cells and organs. In my mind's eye I had a vision of a five-year-old girl wearing a black and white marine cut-style dress with pink material on the chest. I shook my head to clear my vision but the image grew bigger and the details of the dress became clearer. I had no idea what it was or why I was seeing it. When we finished the session, I gave Mely this feedback. Most clients understand the meaning and significance behind my visions. In most cases they are spiritual messages. Well, Mely didn't know what it was about either. We wrapped up the session and she went home feeling lighter and happier. Later that afternoon she rang to tell me she had asked her mother about the dress, describing its colour and style. Her mother said she had made that dress when she was five years old and that Mely never took it off, not even to get it washed.

I was still working at my other part-time job as a casino croupier. This was where I had met Jean, who worked at the staff canteen. She told me that since her last treatment and the uncovering of the dress story, Mely had become warm and loving again, just like in the old days. The message of the dress was a simple healing tool and a reminder of the beautiful relationship that once existed between a mother and daughter.

Mely and Jean's situation is an example of emotional healing. These are simple words, but when emotional disturbances become toxic they affect our health and relationships with others. If this is not recognised early and dealt with it can have serious consequences, such as excessive grief or sadness leading to lung imbalances. This happened to my mother, as the sadness she endured weakened her lungs. Her constant worries also weakened her heart, which eventually took her life. On the plus side I took my daughter to the family home in the Philippines for the first time and she had the opportunity to meet with her grandmother, which provided some good and lasting memories for her. However, this was to be the first and last time...

As promised, I will now elaborate on the experience I had as a five-year-old (see: Journey to Wellness) when, on a Sunday afternoon, my father came home intoxicated. It is normal for children to try to make their parents happy. As my daughter grew up, her soul always found ways to please me and her dad. All the marvellous things I thought I was doing to protect my father's beautiful garden – such as intercropping corn with watermelon – made my inner child feel hurt and confused. I had thought I was doing him a favour by keeping the chickens away, as unripe watermelon was very attractive to them. I thought I was being kind and helpful walking around with a makeshift tin shaker filled with little stones. I wanted to deter the chickens and make a trail, killing the watermelon vines that I chose to walk on.

It never occurred to me that I was damaging the whole plantation. This, of course, made my father angry. In his eyes, I had failed, which evoked a physical violent reaction from him and caused me to pass out. Upon regaining consciousness, I noticed my little brother trying to wake me. He was three years old and possibly thought that I was just falling asleep. Since then my adventurous mind filled with fear. I was confused because the kindness I had offered had brought harm to me. I had kept this incident to myself, and could not tell anyone – not even my mother – for fear of escalating the chaos in the household. My mother was very protective to all of her children, employing her own methods of discipline, which were the opposite to that of my father's, who was stern and demonstrative. This produced conflict between my parents. I always acted as a peacemaker; being a Libran kid, I suppose that says it all. I was always frightened of my dad and, as I grew older, I felt anger towards him. Helpless as I was, all I could do was suppress my emotions and learn to pretend that everything was okay. I had observed this practice from my mother and applied it until such time when I forgave him prior to his passing.

Three

CHAKRA HEALING – OPENING ENERGETIC CENTRES

'Self-love requires you to be honest about your current choices and thought patterns and undertake new practices that reflect self worth.'

– CAROLINE KIRK

Some Eastern cultures describe the energy sources in our bodies as chakras, which are distinguished by their own corresponding colours and symbols. It is said that there are seven centres of spiritual power in the human body. In a simplistic way, I think of them as 'antennae' or 'aerials' picking up signals from the divine source and the universe so that your whole being can maintain balance. If you wish to know more, this super power is easy to learn and can take you to a higher level in the fifth dimension.

Each chakra governs and relates to a specific organ and part of the body. Suffering from long illnesses can indicate the depletion or imbalance of your chakras and could require deeper healing on a spiritual level. The chakra system originated in India between 1500 and 500 BC in the oldest text called the Vedas (the Book of Knowledge), the most sacred scriptures of Hinduism and the oldest text on the planet.

What follows is a brief explanation of chakra positions relative to our body and the corresponding associations and colours. The following sources can also be found on my website.

Since learning about chakra energy my outlook on life has changed. As this has helped me, my hope is that it will help you too. Many are still unaware of chakra energy, yet I find it one of the keys to getting the utmost out of life. You can start healing your own chakras by meditating. Visualise each symbol and colour and imagine closed petals opening as you perform the process of chakra healing. It is best to start at the root chakra. This is a foundation, grounding you as you work your way up to the crown. You can also seek help from chakra healers, who will help you recognise which chakras need healing. When I perform chakra healing, my clients tell me they can feel and sense the energy rushing along their entire body. On my website are free audio files that will help you. To find them, visit www.healingmydivineself.com.au and click the Self-Help tab.

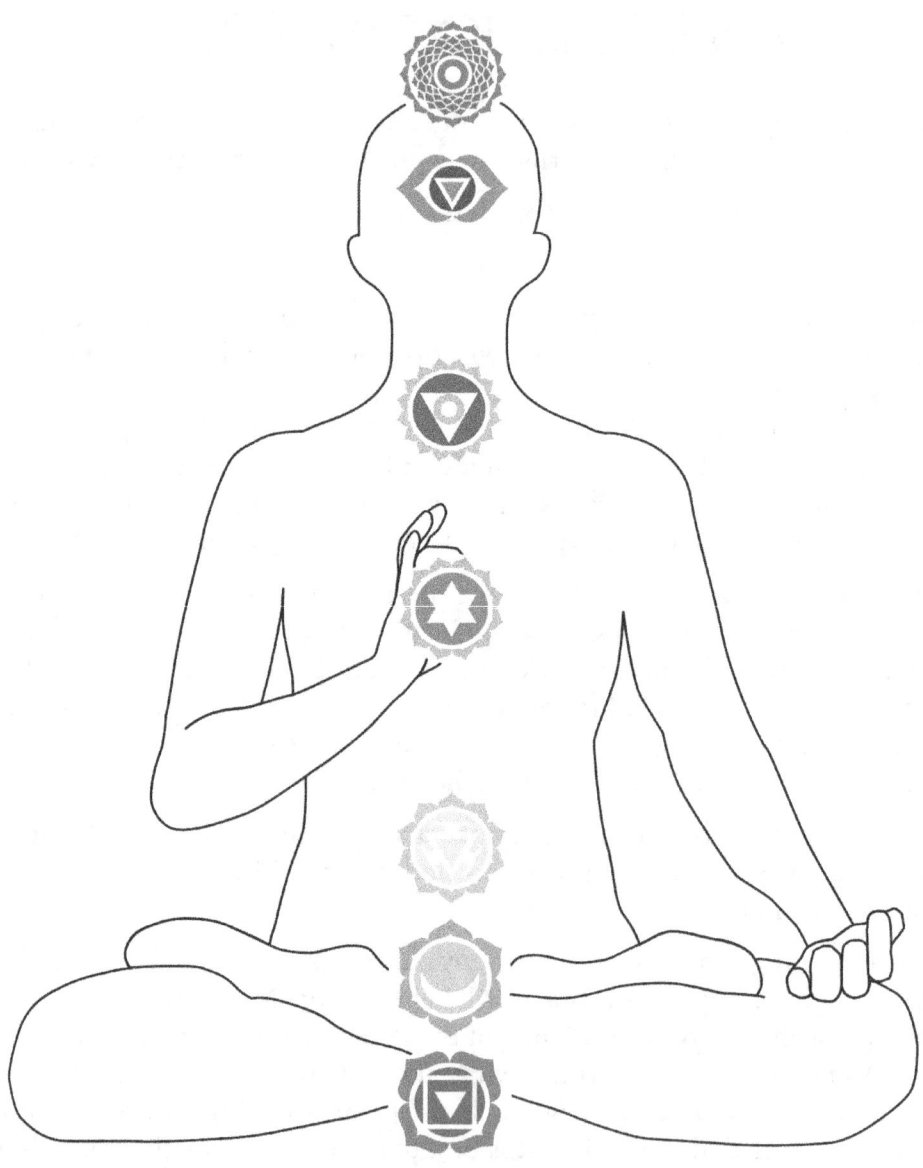

The Root Chakra

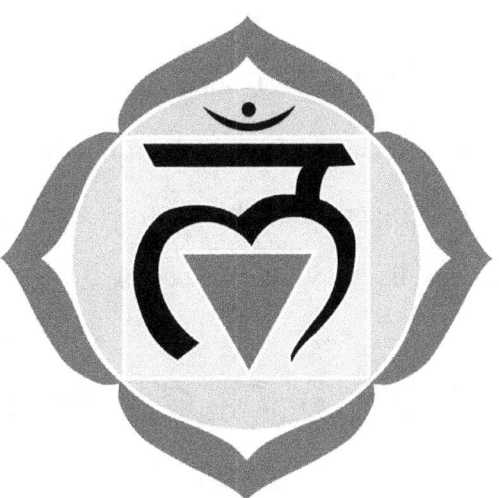

Mulhadra Root Chakra

The root chakra Mulādhāra (referred to in English as 'root support') is symbolised by a lotus with four petals and the colour red. This centre is located at the base of the spine in the coccygeal region. It is said to relate to the gonads and the adrenal medulla and is responsible for the fight-or-flight response. It is all about feeling.

Grounded Muladhara is related to instinct, security, survival, finances, food and shelter, and basic human potentiality. Physically, Muladhara governs sexuality; mentally, it governs stability; emotionally, it governs sensuality; while spiritually it governs a sense of security. Muladhara also relates to the sense of smell.

Red relates to self-awareness. It is the area of survival and stability and your place on this earth. The colour red provides the power from the earth and gives energy on all levels. It connects us to our physical body. Everything that is to be commenced needs the life vitality of red.

- **Positive aspects of red:** Security, courage, strength of will, pioneering.

- **Negative aspects of red:** Insecurity, self-pity, aggression, fear.

Healing Foods

- Red-coloured foods, like beetroots.
- Hot spices, like red cayenne peppers and Tabasco sauce.
- Vegetables from the ground, like potatoes and carrots.
- Animal proteins, like red meat and eggs.

The Sacral Chakra

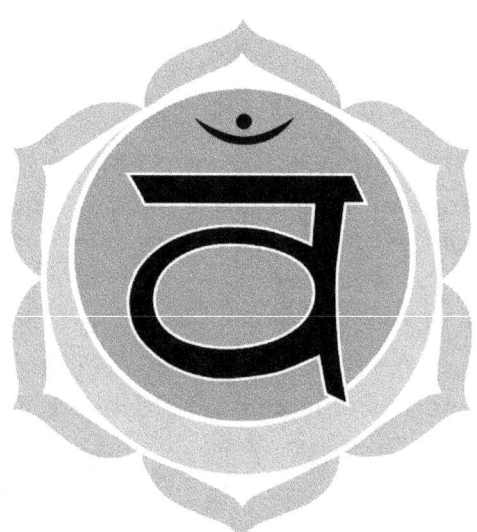

Svadhishthana Sacral Chakra

The sacral chakra Svādhiṣṭhāna (referred to in English as 'one's own base') is symbolised by a white lotus. Within this lotus is a crescent moon with six vermilion or orange petals. This chakra is located in the sacrum and is considered to correspond to the testes or ovaries, which produce the various sex hormones involved in the reproductive cycle. Svādhiṣṭhāna is also more generally considered to be related to the genitourinary system and the adrenals. The key issues involving Svādhiṣṭhāna are relationships, violence, addictions, basic emotional needs and pleasure. Physically, Svādhiṣṭhāna governs reproduction; mentally, it governs creativity; emotionally, it governs joy; and spiritually, it governs enthusiasm and our ability to accept others and new experiences. Orange is the colour of success and relates to self-respect. It gives us the freedom to be ourselves and helps us expand our interests and activities. Orange brings joy to our workday and strengthens our appetite for life! It is the best emotional stimulant, connecting us to our senses and helping to remove inhibitions. It also makes us independent and social.

- Positive aspects of orange: Sociable, creative, joyous, independence.
- Negative aspects of orange: Withdrawn, destructive, despondent, overdependence.

Healing Food

- Orange-coloured foods, like oranges, pumpkin, tangerines and nuts.

The Solar Plexus Chakra

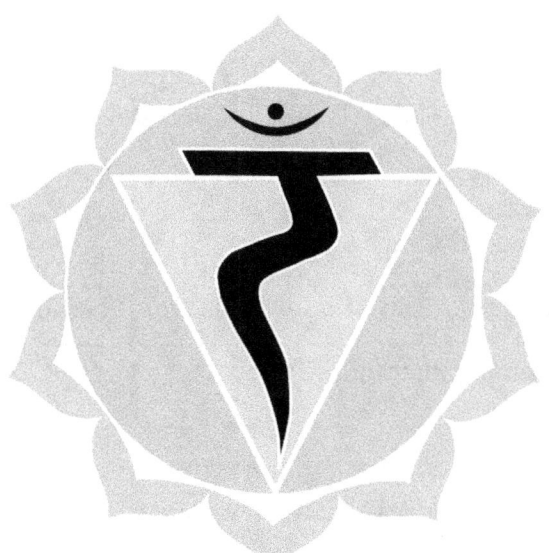

Manipura Solar Plexus Chakra

The solar plexus chakra Maṇipūra (known in English as 'jewel city') is symbolised by a downward pointing triangle with ten petals. Maṇipūra is believed to correspond to Islets of Langerhans, which are groups of cells in the pancreas, as well as the outer adrenal glands and the adrenal cortex. These play a valuable role in digestion, the conversion of food matter into energy for the body.

The colour that corresponds to Maṇipūra is yellow. Key issues governed by Maṇipūra are issues of personal power, fear, anxiety, opinion formation, introversion, and transition from simple or base emotions to complex ones. Physically, Maṇipūra governs digestion; mentally, it governs personal power; emotionally, it governs expansiveness; and spiritually, it governs all matters of growth. Yellow is a creative colour and relates to self-worth, how we feel about ourselves and how we feel others perceive us. This is the area of the personality, the ego and the intellect. Yellow gives us clarity of thought, increases awareness and stimulates interest and curiosity. Yellow energy is related to the ability to perceive and understand. It connects us to our mental self and our ability to be confident and feel in control of our lives. It is also called the power chakra.

- Positive aspects of yellow: Confidence, alertness, optimism, good sense of humour.

- Negative aspects of yellow: Feelings of inferiority, over analytical, sarcasm, pessimism.

Healing Foods

- Yellow-coloured foods, like corn.

- Grains and fibre, granola and whole wheat bread.

- Peppermint and chamomile tea.

The Heart Chakra

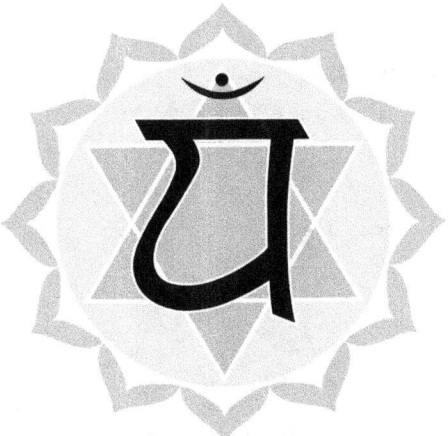

Anahata Heart Chakra

The heart chakra Anāhata (known in English as 'unstuck') is symbolised by a circular flower with twelve green petals called the heart-mind (wisdom). Within it is a yantra, the geometrical patterns of two intersecting triangles, which form a hexagram. This symbolises a union of the male and female. Anāhata is related to the thymus, located in the chest. The thymus is an element of the immune system and is part of the endocrine system. It is the site of maturation of the T cells, which are responsible for fending off disease. It may be adversely affected by stress.

Anāhata is related to the colours green or pink. Key issues involving Anāhata include complex emotions, compassion, tenderness, unconditional love, equilibrium, rejection and wellbeing. Physically, Anāhata governs circulation; emotionally, it governs unconditional love for the self and others; mentally, it governs passion; and spiritually it governs devotion. When balanced, we are able to give love and nurture ourselves. Green helps to relax muscles, nerves and thoughts; cleanse and balance our energy; and give feelings of renewal, joy, inner peace and harmony. Green connects us to unconditional love and is used for balancing our whole being.

- Positive aspects of green: Compassion, generosity, harmony, balance, love.

- Negative aspects of green: Indifference, jealousy, misery, bitterness.

Healing Food

- Green-coloured foods, such as leafy vegetables, kale, spinach and green tea.

The Throat Chakra

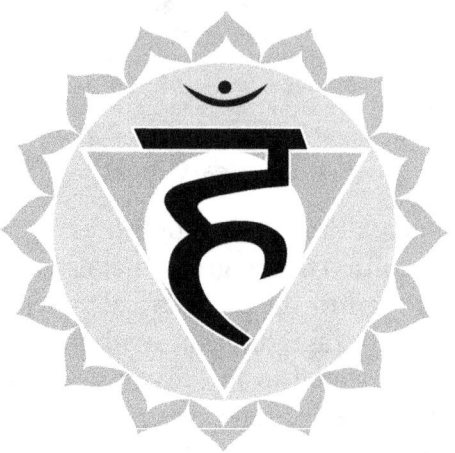

Vishuddha Throat Chakra

The throat chakra Viśuddha (known in English as 'especially pure') is depicted as a silver crescent within a white circle with sixteen pale blue or turquoise petals.

Viśuddha relates to communication and growth through self-expression. This chakra's parallel is the thyroid, a throat gland which produces the hormone responsible for growth and maturation. Physically, Viśuddha governs communication; emotionally, it governs independence; mentally, it governs fluent thought; and spiritually, Viśuddha governs a sense of security.

Blue is the spiritual colour that relates to self-expression, the ability to communicate with our feelings, the spirit of truth and purpose, and secrecy. This is a mentally relaxing colour. Blue has a pacifying effect on the nervous system and brings great relaxation. It is ideal for treating sleep problems and hyperactive children.

Blue connects us to holistic thought and gives us wisdom and clarity, enhancing our communication and speech.

- Positive aspects of blue: Loyal, trustworthy, tactful, calm.
- Negative aspects of blue: Unfaithful, untrustworthy, self-righteous, cold.

Healing Food

- Juices, teas and all types of fruits, especially blueberries.

Third Eye Chakra

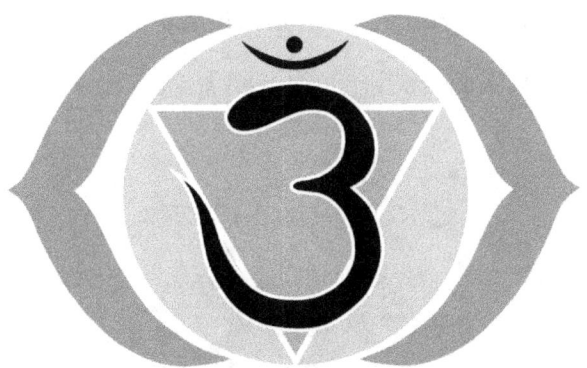

Ajna Third Eye Chakra

The third eye chakra Ājñā (known in English as 'command') is symbolised by a lotus with two petals, and corresponds to the colours indigo or deep blue, though it is traditionally described as white. It is at this point that the two-side nadis Ida (yoga) and Pingala are said to terminate and merge with the central channel Sushumna, signifying the end of duality, the characteristic of being dual (e.g. light and dark, or male and female). Indigo relates to self-responsibility – being responsible for one's own life, responsible to oneself to follow the soul's path and needs, and the trusting of one's own intuition. It gives us the ability to see things from a 'higher' viewpoint, rather than doing things purely for the satisfaction of the ego or one's material comfort.

The indigo energy connects us to our unconscious self and gives us the experience of being part of the whole universe. It strengthens intuition, imagination, psychic powers and increases dream activity and the ability to make decisions.

- Positive aspects of indigo: Highly intuitive, faithful, clear-sighted, orderly mind.
- Negative aspects of indigo: Inability to trust intuition, scattered mind, inconsiderate, blinkered vision.

Healing Food

- Purple-coloured fruits, like grapes and blueberries.
- Dark chocolate, lavender, flavoured spices, cinnamon or tea.

Crown Chakra

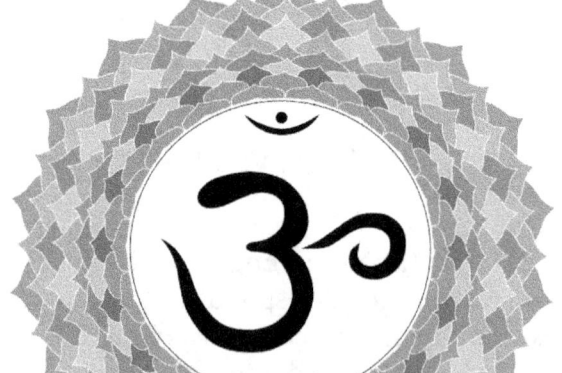

Sahasrara Crown Chakra

The crown chakra Sahasrāra (known in English as 'thousand-petalled') is generally considered the state of pure consciousness, within which there is neither object nor subject. When the Kundalini energy rises to this point it unites with the male Shiva energy and a state of liberating Samadhi is attained.

Symbolised by a lotus with one thousand multi-coloured petals (but often seen as a violet blossom) it is located either at or above the crown of the head. Sahasrāra is represented by the colour white and corresponds to issues such as inner wisdom and the death of the body.

Violet relates to self-knowledge and spiritual awareness. It is the union with our higher self, with spirituality and our higher consciousness. Disease can cause an imbalance of energy in this chakra (i.e. either too much or too little). The violet energy connects us to our spiritual self, guidance, wisdom and inner strength, inner and outer beauty and pure bliss. It purifies our thoughts and feelings, giving us inspiration in all undertakings and enhancing artistic talent and creativity.

- Positive aspects of violet: A reverence for life, self-searching in the service of others, idealism, an ability to see the appropriate route for the benefit of the higher self.

- Negative aspects of violet: No concern for others, feelings of superiority, lack of contact with reality.

Healing Foods

Since the crown chakra represents our spiritual connection to our surroundings, this chakra does not benefit from healing foods. The crown chakra is more likely to benefit from breathing clean and fresh air and sunshine.

Observing my physical energy, moods and emotions every day helps me recognise which chakras I need to work on. Understanding your chakra energy can help you recognise the layers of blockages that prevent you from living the life that you were meant to live. Chakra energy is your antenna connecting you to the universe. It is therefore important to be conscious about the way you feel as the universal vibration and attraction unconsciously responds to your energy operation.

When I studied chakra, I became calmer and more at peace in my life. This eased my negative emotions, such as anger, which subsequently relaxed my physical body, allowing it to repair damage and rejuvenate cells and related organs. When closed, my root and base prevented me from accepting compliments. This also prevented me from accepting my divine self. I was less grounded and my mind was often lost in imagination and I thought often about negative past events. I now know it was a waste of my time dwelling on the past, re-energising it over and over again, daydreaming of one thing or another and jeopardising my focus. Since healing my chakras, I have mostly overcome negative thinking. I now allow myself to explore without self-criticism, self-doubt or self-consciousness. Grounding myself opened me to accepting who I am and what am I here to be.

I also discovered I had the capacity to enjoy sex, which had previously never held the slightest importance to me. My sexual experience was only pain and discomfort. Twenty years ago, I was part of a group of young mothers who had coffee together once a week after dropping our children off at school. The friends would share their sexual stories and joke around, but I was reticent to share and felt uncomfortable. In my time, sex was not really to be explored. We were never allowed to mention it back home, so sitting and listening to their sex stories confused me. I wondered what was so wonderful about it as they enthused about how a glass of wine enhanced their sexual performance. Chakra healing made me so much more in control of my life.

Four

THE ANGELS – HEALING LIGHTS

'To receive divine guidance, become still and listen to the intuitive nudges. The way becomes clear when you do.'

– **Dean Jackson**

My inner guides guided me to integrate healing angels in this book for chakra healing. Archangels carry a unique colour vibration that corresponds to particular chakras and represents specific virtues. They have different tasks and can be called upon to help you heal your chakras. In my healing sessions I call upon the highest and best archangels to guide me. Angels have been mentioned all over the world in different spiritual traditions and are known by different names. While writing this book, I asked for guidance to find the most suitable and comprehendible information sources for my readers. I was guided to an online course where I connected with Kyle Gray, author and expert angel communicator. Kyle is a mentor who runs several online courses – one of which is Connecting with Your Angels. When loving spirits see us struggling they hang around, waiting to show us the solutions.

For example, the healing energy of Archangel Raphael can be felt in hospitals by sick people. Angels can assist us in so many ways, helping us find peace. However, the only way they can is if we welcome them. We must acknowledge their presence and invite their guidance. They operate at a high vibration frequency. Therefore we need to raise our vibration close to theirs in order to connect on a deeper level. Loving ourselves raises our vibration. As Kyle Gray's book explains, there are three angel hierarchy levels, which are broken down into spheres. Each sphere contains three different types of angel and angels of a particular type are known as a choir. To make things easier: there are nine choirs of angels organised in three spheres. Each choir has an overall purpose, though there will be specific angels in each choir that have special gifts to offer. All angels have one true focus: love, peace and harmony for the whole universe.

Most of us are probably only familiar with our guardian angels, which are the angels on the third sphere. This is because some of their roles go beyond Earth. Kyle Gray explains that the spheres of angels all stand around the heart of God. In the centre of the spheres lies God's energy, which is sent out through thoughts. These thoughts create angels. The angels then look back at God and sing His praises and the praises of all creation. This expression of love radiates love energy.

The First Spheres are:

- The seraphim are the highest choir of angels. These angels, whose name means 'burning ones', are beautiful flames of universal love. Some describe them as having six or eight wings. If there is an angelic government it would be made up of the seraphim. They are known for the beautiful praises which they sing of God. These bring energetic shifts and waves of healing to the whole universe.

- The cherubim are the choir of angels that created cherubs. These divine angels are very knowledgeable about the universe. In fact, their name means 'fullness of knowledge'. They are God's record keepers and are closely connected to the Akashic records, a chronicle of every event that has ever happened in the whole of creation.

- The thrones are angels seen as wheels of light. The word 'throne' relates to the seat on which God sits, although God also goes beyond. These angels are in control of universal shifts of consciousness. They work closely with the planet Earth as it moves into a greater awareness of spirit and love.

The Second Spheres are:

- Dominions regulate the role of every angel, apart from those in the first sphere. Their name means 'lordships' and they are figures of authority. These angelic beings oversee international affairs. They are wonderful to call on for help in international situations, including conflicts and disasters.

- Virtues are the angels who look after the flow of nature. They ensure that the world is balanced according to the natural laws and bring blessings to individual countries. Their name means 'strongholds' and it is believed that these angels weave the natural flow of life force.

- Powers are the race of angels that encourage us to remember there is a better way. Their whole purpose is to end conflict, destruction and war – whether within your own self-struggle or in general. They are made of pure compassion and send waves of light to the world, especially to those who are trying to push the destruct button on our beautiful planet. They can protect us when we call on them, especially if we are asking them to support us on a national level.

THE THIRD SPHERES ARE:

- Principalities are the angels who protect spirituality, including spiritual texts. Their name means 'rulers' and they have a strong connection with world leaders and activists who want to make this world a better place. These angels help reveal spiritual truths in science so that we can understand the divinity of our creation even more.

- Archangels are the boss angels. They are in charge of all the guardian angels who look after Earth, its inhabitants and their journey of spiritual growth. Archangels are a magnificent group of angels and are ready and willing to work with us at any time. Everyone knows who they are in heaven and knows their amazing gifts and talents. There are thousands of archangels. We know more of them than others. Divine Guidance, authored by Doreen Virtue, can help you identify more angels and archangels.

- The final choir of angels is the most exciting one. This includes our own very dear guardian angels, the healing angels and the angels of planet Earth. This choir is the one we direct access to when we tune in to angels. They are what this chapter is all about. When we send our thoughts to heaven, the angel who is best able to help us will leave this choir and come directly to us. If they feel they need the support of a higher angel, they will go to them and work together. This beautiful thought can keep us in a higher vibration. When we speak to Heaven, all we need to say is 'angels' because there are so many out there who can help us. When working with clients I call upon their guardian angel to communicate with me in order to assist in healing their divine self.

I enlist the help of the following angels during my chakra healing sessions.

Root Chakra

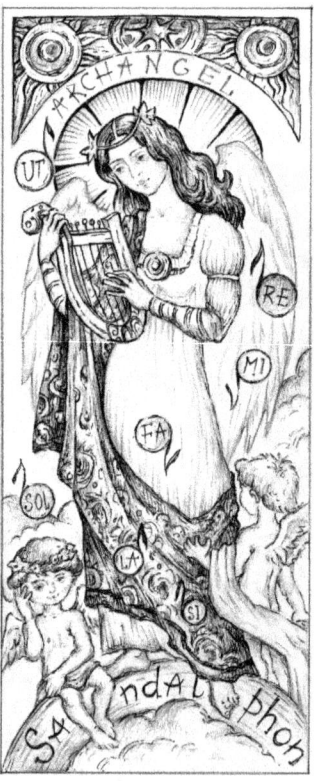

Sandalphon

Sandalphon stands for courage, silence and knowledge. She possesses what is called 'materia' or 'chaos', which is energy that is both active and passive, a duality that can create physical. She is also the archangel linked to music and will guide you if you play the right things. She wants to teach people how to feel good, how to speak in a positive tone, and how to create sound energies. She can make your words and actions gentle and smooth, but still powerful. She also determines the sex of a newborn baby, so is the one to pray to before you get pregnant if you want a boy or girl. She also says that we must create our own lives as nobody else will do it for us. We may even find our truths and beliefs. Find the red thread, the love beyond reason, and take it in your hand. Follow step by step to make sense and find alignment.

Sandalphon's appearance is so high that she can reach from Earth to Heaven. Her aura has a healing and soothing that helps your kundalini energy, the energy that sits dormant in the first chakra at the base of the spine. This energy is released during orgasm through the second chakra when trying to create a child. The kundalini energy is also often released during life-threatening situations. People gain super-human strength to save love ones. For example, a mother may lift a car to save her child. Her kundalini is released, giving her the power to do what she needs to do.

Sacral Chakra

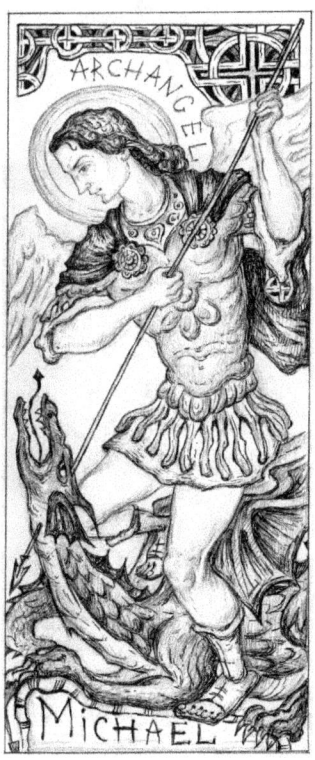

Archangel Michael

Ample angels wait for us to call upon them to heal our divine selves. I call upon these archangels for healing and clearing base chakras. Some people are known to be naturally generous while others have trouble receiving. Archangel Michael can chop the chords of negative energy, removing and releasing you from negative emotional entanglement and negative entities. You can also ask Archangel Gabriel and Archangel Raphael for healing and protecting or ask them to empower you with courage, confidence, strength, vitality and self-esteem.

Solar Plexus Chakra

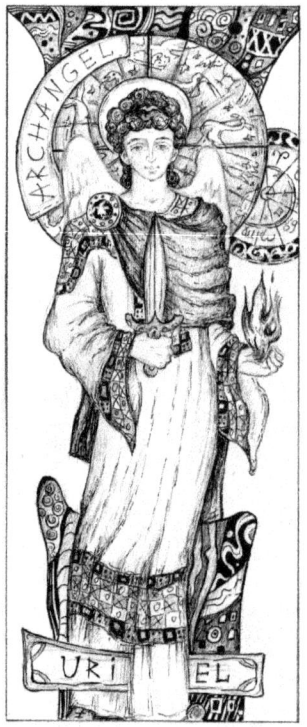

Archangel Uriel

I call on Archangel Uriel for chakra healing. He is a link to the higher realms that can illuminate your soul purpose, lift your burdens and ignite your intuition. He is often depicted with an open hand holding a flame that brings light to all souls. This light can fuel your passion and bring insights and understanding. Archangel Uriel transmutes all lower energies and emotions into the higher vibrations of spiritual understanding, love and compassion. He can also elevate your psychic senses and open you to clairvoyance and universal consciousness.

Call upon Archangel Uriel when you need help with intuition, alchemy, astrology, esoteric wisdom, or divine guidance. I have also known Uriel to help with weather balance. When my rain water tank is getting low I call the rain from him and, in a few hours or a day, rain clouds start forming. Once in the Philippines the weather bureau of meteorology reported that a typhoon was just three hours away from hitting our village. My brother and I called Archangel Uriel and asked that the typhoon be diverted somewhere else. Suddenly the strong wind eased off and became calm.

Heart Chakra

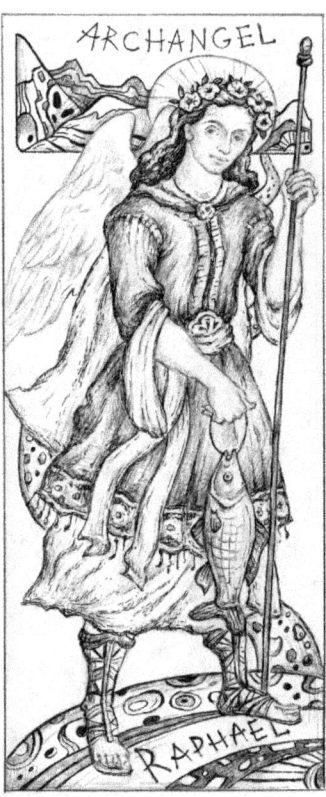

Archangel Raphael

Archangel Raphael is the one I call for heart chakra healing. He is the healing angel of miracles who restores your physical, emotional, financial and spiritual wellbeing. Embodying the energies of unconditional love and compassion, he can bring healing to any situation or circumstance. He can even heal Earth itself. You can call upon this healing angel to assist you in forgiving yourself and others. Archangel Raphael can also help you let go of emotional and physical toxins, negative relationships, addictions, recovery, health concerns, weight loss, and healing the planet and its inhabitants.

Throat Chakra

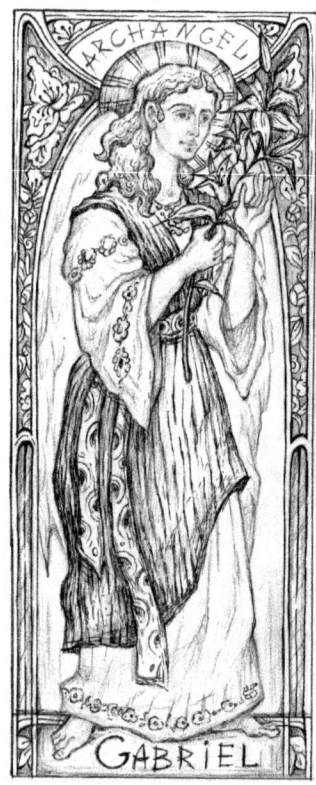

ARCHANGEL GABRIEL

Archangel Gabriel, whose name means 'messenger of God', can help you communicate the truth about who you are, where you have been and your inner vision. He is the most powerful of all angelic messengers and will work with you to clear your throat chakra of any blockages. This archangel will help you reclaim your personal power, empowering you with gifts, skills and talents. It isn't necessary to speak your truth to anyone but yourself. Your throat chakra is the centre of all communication, whether you speak silently to yourself or aloud to the people around you. When you hold on to something you really feel the need to express because you are afraid of the consequences or how someone will perceive you, you swallow fear energy. This is then collected and stored in your throat chakra, causing your energy to be blocked. When your throat chakra is blocked with fear you disempower yourself. However, Archangel Gabriel can help you embrace your authenticity with conviction and compassion.

THIRD EYE CHAKRA

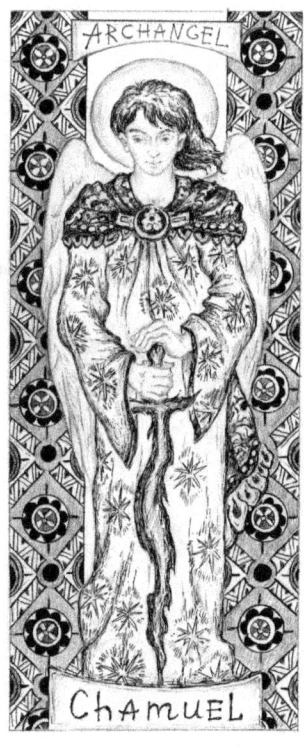

Archangel Chamuel

I call upon Archangel Chamuel for third eye chakra. Using his omniscient vision, this archangel can see the connection between everyone and everything. You can call upon him anytime you would like to see your life from a higher perspective. He can assist you with all you seek, including finding the right resources to fulfil your soul's purpose or clarity for your direction. He is known for peaceful relationship and can help you find your soulmate and resolve conflict with others. If you are looking with inner peace, he can help you find the spiritual meaning in any challenging situation.

Crown Chakra

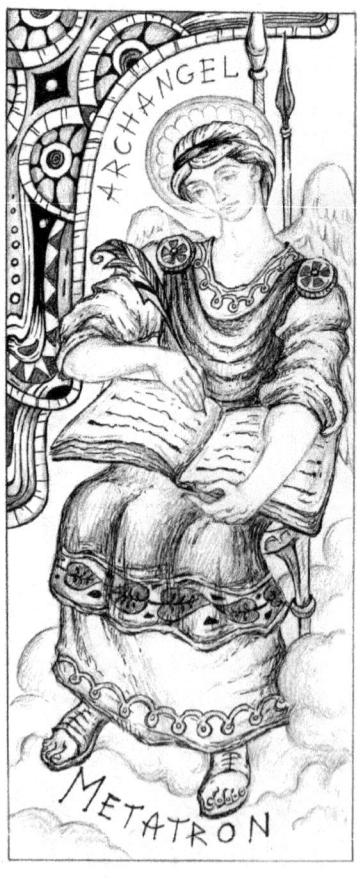

Archangel Metatron

Metatron is the highest level and the first manifestation of the infinite stream of energy emanating from the Father/Mother. He is a seraph angel, but he is also the highest cherub and manages everything with his right hand, which is called Michael. His left hand is his female part. Her name is Sandalphon, though some call her Gabriel. Metatron also has the title of archangel. Author Philip Alexander said that Metatron is best to be invoked on Sundays, when the energy sphere from Keter, the planet Pluto and the crown chakra are working perfectly together.

Five

ENERGY BLOCKS – FINDING ENERGY BLOCKS

> 'People were created to be loved, things are created to be used, the reason why the world is in chaos is because things are being loved and people are being used.'
>
> – DALAI LAMA

At the age of thirteen I was a tomboy. I worked equally with men, climbing coconut trees and preparing the field for rice planting. There was no man's job I could not do. Low and behold I became my father's favourite child. On weekends my older brothers and I rode on the buffalos as they fed, tediously ensuring they only ate grass and not the rice plant. Time went on and, by the age of fourteen, I had either forgotten or accepted the violent actions inflicted on me by my father when I was five years old.

Our father had this routine where he would go to town to watch cockfighting – the cruellest entertainment for people to enjoy on a Sunday afternoon. I never really enjoyed it when I had a chance to watch it. My father would meet up with his friends for a drink then come home. He was getting older then and, because of illness and a near death experience, had started to slow down his drinking. He was not supposed to drink anymore but he still did.

At that time, my fear of him was subsiding and I was a lot closer to my brothers than to my older sisters. I somehow developed a shield of protection from my physical abuse experience. I appeared to be the toughest person at school and in college. No one dared to mess with me. I became less kind, demanding and somewhat abusive to anyone who crossed my path. One of my sisters called me the black sheep in the family. The anger that had replaced fear was mounting and when I got married I carried on the cycle I'd inherited from my mother: not to marry a person who loved alcohol. Unfortunately the man I married, my husband, had a fondness for drinking. However, we managed to stay together for fifteen years, arguing often until we both ran out of patience. At that time most of my energy was spent strategising to smoothen our lives for our daughter. After separating from husband my daughter and I moved from one friend's home to another on weekends. My husband and I had difficulties being in the same place and communication was getting difficult. He claimed my English was getting harder to understand. I refused to communicate with him while he was intoxicated; my English as a second language had never been a problem when he was sober. Life became very stressful and its lack of meaning lowered our self-esteem. I didn't want our daughter to see what I'd seen when I was young. Because of our situation at that time I could visualise my daughter continuing the trend to the third generation. The cycle of unhealthy family situation was not to be condoned anymore, which prompted my decision to separate. The fear and anger that I locked into my DNA level had never been acknowledged at that time. I was still avoiding my responsibilities and kept attracting people of the same category, which I did not know until I studied forensic energy and chakra healing.

I was never aware that our emotions affect our physical bodies until I became ill. Peter, my next partner, had to call a doctor in the middle of the night a few times because I felt unbearable pain in my upper stomach. When I consulted medical specialists, they ran me through scans but never found anything. They suggested more examinations and performed keyhole surgery with a camera inside my stomach, so they could thoroughly examine my problem. I was already a part-time therapist at that time, doing reflexology and aromatherapy. I appreciated that these medical professionals were doing their best to help, but my concern was that in the meantime I would be dosed up on drugs. If they could not see the problem through a scan, what then? This time I was not prepared to undertake further procedures. I decided to take care of my pain myself (notice 'my pain' – words also used by most of my clients). I had no idea how to resolve this but told them I would try to find the solution. They suggested for me to take Nexium medication for gastroesophageal reflux diseases to minimise the pain. Taken three times a day with no dietary adjustments, it helped a little. But then the pain hit again big time and I had to increase the dose of the medication. I also altered my diet to include only steamed food. This caused me to rapidly lose weight – and I didn't have much to lose, as I was always a petite person. It was physically apparent that I had health problems. My friends would joke that I needed to eat more to fatten myself up. Many of them did not really know what I been through and looking and feeling unwell was not really did not reflect well on my therapy business.

I decided to stop the medication and take care of my own health. While in town, I spontaneously went to the book store, not really sure what I needed. In the health section I found Dr Sandra Cabot's book *Raw Juices Can Save Your Life* sticking halfway out of the shelf. I immediately experienced a kind of take-me-home attraction. It wasn't the same powerful feeling I experienced with my reflexology book; this time it was more of an attraction. Checking the table of contents I noticed the recipes were listed alphabetically by raw fruits and vegetables. The book claimed stomach pain was related to gall bladder – the liver's partner, according to Chinese medicine. For relief, I needed to make a mixture of celery, carrots and apple. But first I would need a juicer, which I got on the way home, no mucking around. I religiously made juices at least three times a day for a week. Peter was in charge of the weekly shopping and made sure that our fridge never ran out of those three things. He was very supportive when it came to my health and never hesitated to try everything he could to help in a natural way. We were of the same mind and hoped to find natural solutions using whole foods rather than medication. I concede that in some cases medication helps, but there always seems to be side effects that go with it. When I had painful attacks Peter let me press my solar plexus on his shoulder and bounce around while walking. My weight must have been very uncomfortable for him. He had to walk around with me on his shoulder, like he was carrying a bag of potatoes. However, this seemed to relieve the pain slightly. It was the kind of pain that you will trade anything and everything just to be rid of it. My prayers to escape that painful misery were answered by juicing. This made me more interested in natural remedies. I learnt that eating more herbs, fruits and vegetables would support my immune system, allowing my body to repair itself. I now include this information in my healing sessions.

My pain eventually started to subside. I started eating a lot more without fear that food could trigger the pain. Every night Peter would leave slices of apple, celery and carrot on my bedside in case I experienced discomfort in the middle of the night. It was a little ritual. It did experience pain every now and then, usually, I noted, when I indulged in fatty foods or sweets. This was the most common trigger.

After five years, I was pain free. It was all thanks to Dr Cabot's book. It really saved my life. My experience of going through this and managing to heal myself gave me the idea to write *Healing My Divine Self*. I chose to empower myself and not give up before my time. Our challenges could be a gift to remind other earth walkers that they are not alone. The divine source is unlimited. We just need to open our hearts and minds so that we can hear them and be guided in the direction of happiness and peace.

At this time, I did not know what energy blocks were. I knew in a scientific sense that energy is everything and everything is energy, but had no clue that it affected every situation – even finances. I have always had a reasonable job and always managed to afford most things that my daughter and I needed. We were even able to send some help back to my siblings in the Philippines. I intend to save up for the rainy days or for just the sake of saving. I noticed my pattern of money handling; no matter how much I earned from my two jobs, by the end of the week my finances always return to their starting point. As soon as I save few dollars another reason arises for my savings to leak out. I remember I got paid $400 for a treatment from a client who comes in every week and pays me at the end of the month. While I was holding the money I asked myself what I would do with this money. The universe must have been right in my face listening as always because my daughter called me crying thirty minutes later. She told me our two eleven-month-old puppies had gotten into the shed and climbed up the garden shelves. They'd gotten into a box of snail bait that I had hidden away. Obviously they'd thought the box of snail pellets were dog treats. Sadly one of them did not make it. It was the most gorgeous, loving puppy, always full of energy and always hungry. Every time I came home from work I would find her falling asleep in self-feeder bowl, eating puppy biscuits. She was getting so fat that we had to eliminate the self-feeder and start giving them food at feeding time only. Fortunately, the other puppy survived. My daughter got him to the vet just in time with her boyfriend, who soon after became her husband. This cheeky puppy is beloved by my clients and the whole neighbourhood.

Analysing all of these cycles of life, I recall one very significant piece of wisdom my mother told to me when I was very young. We were having an afternoon snack and I kept asking for more. My mother told me there was no more, leaving me with this memory that remains encrypted in my brain. She said, 'When you grow up, study well so you can always get a good job that pays you well. That way you'll be able to buy food and everything you want and wish to have in your life.' It did not sound that important but it explains my financial pattern until it was resolved and corrected through forensic healing.

Part of my job involves observing every client that comes to see me and respecting the way they are. One day a lady came to talk to me about her painful experience. She was so stuck in her story of owning the pain. For her, it was like a competition; nobody else had it worse than she did. She had seen many practitioners that she thought could help and even learned of the modalities. As a practitioner myself, I am always willing and eager to help anyone who needs my assistance. However, I gleaned from the conversation and her opinions that she was exploring many options and gathering information. It was possible she would move onto the next practitioner and tell them what the previous healer had extolled. As the session progressed I realised she was very lonely and that she had migrated to Australia without her family. Due to her circumstance she was absorbed in her own pain and had no one who could relieve her of her problem. She was not open to opinion and until she was prepared to let go, so to speak, her ailment would always be present. In my opinion, her method of holding onto the pain was preventing her from letting it go. As a practitioner I have found that listening and patiently absorbing information generally reveals a satisfactory outcome. This is what I did in this instance. I advised her that until she was prepared to 'let go' and listen her problem would remain with her.

Two weeks before my daughter's wedding day, my daughter and I went to town to look for a nice pair of shoes. She wanted me to wear something that would match my dressing gown. Being an older person, my choice was not to her taste anymore. But it was her day after all, so she gets her way with all my pleasure. While I was trying these high-heel shoes on I must have twisted myself. Somehow this triggered a little pain in my neck. They were very nice shoes and we still bought them, as my daughter really liked them. I remained quiet and didn't let her know about my discomfort. We later stopped to have something to eat just outside the mall. I could see she was very excited planning the entire event herself. All we can do as family is be there to offer our assistance if it is asked for. However, my daughter and her husband handled everything nicely themselves. I did not want to disappoint her by telling her I might not be able to wear the nice-looking shoes we bought earlier that day. It became especially difficult when she told me she couldn't wait to see me wearing the whole outfit she'd chosen for me for her special day. My neck pain was progressing, but I kept up my enthusiasm. After all, her happiness has always been my happiness ever since she was born. She is the one who taught me how to feel real love, and to offer everything with altruism, which totally changed my whole life. I learnt to love myself so I can love her more.

The pain in my neck was getting worse. Whenever I moved or laughed tension radiated slowly down to my left shoulder. We were supposed to do more shopping as soon as we finished our food, but as I was getting up I could hardly move; I had to ask her to take me home and continue the shopping the next day. When I got home the pain got worse. As my client said, it felt like all my muscles had locked up on me and I was not allowed to do anything.

My client's story brought me back to this agonising similar experience. I was stuck with the pain the whole week and my stress level kept increasing. My daughter's wedding was now very close and I did not want her to feel sad or concerned about my situation. My partner took me to four different practitioners in the space of a week. In the end I just had to lie in bed and surrender. There I was back having my quiet time, connecting with my inner self and learning to meditate. The next day my muscles started to let go. I could slowly move again without the excruciating pain. I continued to go deeper, not questioning it, surrendering to my inner self and the divine. I asked for guidance from the angels who rejoiced with me as my pain starting to subside. I managed to get up for my daughter's wedding, with only a little niggle from my neck whenever I turned too quickly. The only regret was I was not able to wear the beautiful shoes that my daughter had chosen for me, but it was all okay; I did not need to punish myself for that and my daughter was always been understanding. That's a part of her that I really appreciate.

See, my blockage in my neck was my trying to control things that are already beyond my control. For awhile my sister was living with us feeling emotionally vulnerable. I went along with anything she demanded in order to pacify the grief she was experiencing after separating from her husband. However, maintaining the peace became very stressful for me. Against my wishes, she dug out the lawn in my backyard to replace it with a veggie garden. Tensions rose and gathered in my body. My throat chakra was the first to close up. This is because I was not able to express my emotions for fear that I might upset my sister.

Six

FORENSIC ENERGY HEALING REVELATION OF THE HEALING SECRET

'You were born a child of light's wonderful secret… You return to the beauty you have always been.'

– ABERJHANI

Have you ever experienced a sickness from which you were unable to recover? Even visiting multiple doctors and taking different tests gave little to no improvement. This is sometimes referred to as a mystery illness. Sometimes doctors run out of treatment ideas and advise you to live with your affliction. You could even be accused of being a hypochondriac, told your mind is playing games with you, or told to take antidepressants, a medication that will help you deal with life.

As an alternative, try forensic healing, which sometimes reveals that illnesses can stem from emotional or physical blockages. These can often be helped with acupuncture, acupressure, Reiki, or other natural healing modalities. Forensic healing is an energy-healing modality that goes deeper to find the root of an illness.

Maybe you have experienced trauma in your childhood that you cannot remember, or have taken on board beliefs imposed by someone else – for example, from family members, mentors, or teachers. In fact, anyone is capable of influencing you and depriving you of the right to be 'yourself'. Forensic healing combines kinesiology, energy healing, hands-on healing and healing secrets to free the body of pain, stress and unwanted conditions. This healing modality is renowned as the fourth most powerful healing modality in the world. It can balance relationships, stress, financial blocks, health conditions or anything that causes us stress or pain. Forensic healing empowers by providing answers to why some things occur in life. It will also release emotional, spiritual and physical blocks, so that balance and harmony is restored. Often these (mostly) negative beliefs play in the back of our minds on a subconscious level.

This can affect our lives physically, becoming an illness or limitation. They make us feel 'stuck' and unable to live the life of our dreams.

This powerful healing modality was founded and taught by Marisa Russo. My doors of life keep opening to allow in the good things that are unfolding. Being able to communicate with angels and ascended masters was all I needed, but I long to keep studying as I don't yet feel good enough. If I can learn more I will achieve some contentment in life.

Before I had forensic healing in my life, I made many wrong decisions. Ego kept coming on strong, as negative beliefs that were embedded in my DNA level had not yet been cleared. I had to open up and hear the message from the angels. I believe this was arranged divinely as the next door led me to forensic healing. I remembered discussions with my daughter about the choices we make in life. She told me my choice in partners was poor and that I did not seem to find the best one, which is what I deserved. This alarming point prompted me to deeply examine my life situation. I needed concrete information that I could trust to support my beliefs. I struggled a lot. I considered meditation, but I was not a good meditator. Meditating seems to stress me out more – especially long guided sessions. My mind just cannot focus on relaxing. I kept worrying about the bills I had to pay for the next six months instead of focussing on the moment. I realised this after reading Eckhart Tolle's *The Power of Now*.

While studying forensic healing I discovered one of my blockages in my timeline had originated when I was four years old. People somehow perceived me as a troublemaker. When my older sisters or anyone talked negatively about someone behind their back, I would dob them in. Because of this, when others were around me they spoke English so that I wouldn't be able to understand them. I only started learning English when I began school. Once I learned it, though, I became one to watch. A sudden quiet when I entered the room meant they were mouthing off someone but were frightened to do it in front of me. Because of this I subconsciously started to dislike myself. These feelings, combined with my father's physical abuse, took a toll on my self-worth. They also caused me to develop psychological complex concerning males, which made it difficult for me to hold onto a relationship. I thought then that I must keep studying and obtaining more diplomas. Only then would I get back to who I really was and to fulfilling my purpose on Earth.

After forensic healing, I started to feel content. The urge to study subsided and I felt more relaxed and happier. I had let go and meditation became easier. As a practitioner, I now feel more fulfilled in my healing career. Watching women transform after releasing physical pain, traumas and negative beliefs is very rewarding. One client came to unblock her feelings of frustration that had stemmed from her not being able to find a job despite all the training she'd done. At age six her mother had been abusive to her, telling her she wasn't good enough and was hopeless. My client took this abuse and locked it in. Belief in her mother's words had created negative energy and led to my client's new reality.

After clearing all this negative energy, my client felt a lightness in her whole body. She decided to take up meditation to calm her mind and focus on her next aim: manifesting a job. The very next day she called to thank me for the session and told me that someone had given her a free meditation CD. She noticed people were being kinder to her and she felt positive. She also said she could feel that it wouldn't be long before she started working again.

Another beautiful heart-centred lady, a regular client for few years now, loves reflexology and the other healing modalities I incorporate. She says they leave her feeling well and light after a session. When I was learning forensic healing I used to practice on her and discovered some of the reasons behind her behaviour. She appeared to be a very happy person on the outside, but could be very emotional. I did not understand her sensitivity or the random ages that our forensic healing sessions uncovered in her timeline. The sessions helped her sensitivity and emotional issues, and she is now becoming more transparent and more accepting. She believed she already fully loved herself, but the tears that came were a sign of self-pity, which she gradually started to clear.

I remember a lady multiple sclerosis came into my forensic healing class. She had to use a walker as she was unable to balance anymore due to this crippling disease. On the third day she started walking on her own, taking a few steps, and, at the end of the week, she was fully walking around the room, getting her own cup of tea during our breaks. It was an amazing, mind-blowing progress.

When a person is ready and open to let go and release all the layers of negative life pattern and beliefs, the body will then start to incorporate this change and heal itself, a process which is supplemented with naturally grown organic food. A healthy body will do its jobs of supporting your soul for your life purpose. Forensic healing breaks down layers of blockages or doors that were erected because of all the challenges you have gone through in all levels of life – even past lives.

While partnering with another student, I had another mind-blowing experience. We were trying to discover the blocks from our past lives.

They traced all the way back to past generations. I was fascinated by two women who did not know each other from a bar of soap, but who nonetheless felt familiar with each other. During the workshop, everyone received a healing session with our teacher. One of the two women had her turn and cried as she was able to release some of her unwanted issues. As this was happening, the other lady on the set was also crying. None of us understood what was going on. In my mind, I thought she just pitied herself, as our emotions can get affected feeling for others.

As we comforted her we found out that their souls were actually connected from their past lives and were entangled in a similar situation. The unresolved argument from their past lives had never been healed or resolved, so they cleared and released their pain at the same time.

As I am running my workshop for healing my divine self, my workshop organiser shuffles the names of all participants, then instructs them to manifest for the chance to be treated for a day. Manifestation is one topic we cover in the workshop, but we can only take a few participants in the time we have. So to be fair we pick the names of people we could treat with forensic healing and test each one's ability to start manifesting. This way, no one misses out. Actually during healing my divine self I try to teach everyone in the room to heal themselves with the assistance of my energy.

In one class, there were two ladies: one with chronic shoulder pain and the other with debilitating stomach pain. The lady with the shoulder pain described feeling agonising pain whenever she raised her left arm over her head. She had already come to see me for a one-on-one session using other modalities a few months ago and had tried seeing another practitioner. She would get better for a few days and then the pain would slowly creep back. The lady with the stomach pain was in such excruciating pain that she nearly had to cancel her spot at the workshop. I was glad she came to experience her own healing.

Together we performed our group healing, with me assisting everyone regardless of the nature of their discomfort. You must have an open mind if you want to heal energy blocks of any kind. The two ladies managed to heal themselves and gave the most satisfying feedback at the end of the workshop.

Seven

BREAKING THE PATTERNS UNIVERSAL ATTRACTION

'When you complain, you make yourself a victim. Leave the situation, change the situation, or accept it all else its madness.'

– Eckhart Tolle

As the cells in our body transform, energy flow increases will be felt in the autonomic nervous system. Most of us will experience these changes, which occur as our body restructures itself based on messages received from our minds. Electrical sensations will move up and down our whole body. Energies will increase as your thoughts manifest. However, it is good to exercise caution with these thoughts and energies because they will become magnified. As they say, be careful what you wish for because this can cause aches and pains to appear in various parts of the body. Sudden shooting pains in the head or eyes may occur, which could signify that adjustments are being made to your energy field. These adjustments will attune you to different frequencies during cellular transformation. You will learn more about this in the next chapter. The parts of your brain that have been dormant in the past are now being used. This may require some rewiring of brain circuitry, while brain patterns that are no longer functional will be rerouted or healed. As you develop a higher way of thinking and being, you will experience more creative energies and create deeper levels which you can experience through meditation.

As transformation occurs, there may be periods when you feel more anxious and irritable than usual. You may also feel restless, headachy and less able to concentrate. You may also be sensitive to people, sound, smell and your environments, or even experience muscle soreness (particularly in the lower back), joint pain and poor digestion. As your glands are excessively stimulated, your body is in a constant fight-or-flight state, expending resources at tremendous speed.

The transformation process is initiated in the molecular structure of the brain: the house of your mind. The progressive cycle of change is introduced to the rest of the body systems primarily through the cerebral-spinal fluid. From there, it spreads throughout the nervous system in general. This explains the disturbances or sensations felt in the head and spine, such as dizziness, headaches and pressure in the head. It can also cause considerable nervous disruption, sleeplessness, and irregular energy surges. This affects the vagus nerve, the longest cranial nerves, which extend from the brainstem to multiple organs then down to the cranial spinal bone and are vital for our body to function. As our body operates in this sympathetic mood, our muscles continually tense and some of our organs lose their ability to repair and rejuvenate as designed. We need to give ourselves a chance to switch to the parasympathetic –or 'relaxed' – mood, as it's in this state that the body self-heals.

Ignoring your body's signals will slowly weaken your immune system. This will cause new imbalances, which most of us will experience as frustrations, aggression and agitation. Many symptoms are occurring in your body at once. These can include nervous disorders, pressure increases and rising temperatures. It's like a molten mass at the Earth's core, forming a volcano that is ready to erupt at any given time. Only these are explosions of anger and violence. Imbalances in the nervous system can create many disorders, like hypertension, fevers and illnesses. Imbalances in the brainwave system adjust the way thoughts occur.

To put ourselves back to balance, we need natural energy healing. It's a good idea to have more physical contact with the natural world. Try walking with bare feet. Feel the earth and walk on young grass. Going camping is another great way to be close to nature. It can create greater balance in your electromagnetic field. As an experience, I can recommend this to help maintain balance and restore a sense of wellness.

My partner and I went camping in Nelson and spent a couple of days relaxing and reading. It helped us unwind and allowed our bodies to rejuvenate. The etheric body, or 'pure being', acts as a transmitter and receiver for surrounding energies. This takes place in specific energy centres: your body's chakras. Each chakra is directly associated with an endocrine glands. For more information, please refer to the earlier chapter on chakras. If they should fire into the organs and glands, they may inhibit their previously normal functioning. Therefore, we can see the importance of supporting the nervous system at this time as it tries to maintain a state of homeostasis in the body. The body will try to catch up with the increased frequencies of the subtle body. To do this, it will interrupt some of the pathways that these high-intensity impulses travel along. It's just like when someone touches a livewire. They are held there by the current until it is switched off. The body's structures and tissues remain in a stimulated state until these pathways are interrupted by turning off the current. To get a break, we must get back in touch with nature, away from phones, televisions and other negative energy conductors. During this process your body will continue to repair. Systems are being discarded and rebuilt with different structures and compounds, which you can receive through water and air. Food also factors in to electromagnetic reformatting, so make sure you are supporting your body with good-quality food and drink. Avoid junk food. Whole foods with less fat and sugars are best, as your body can efficiently use and identify them.

You will find high levels of excreted proteins in bodily fluids such as urine. The body literally washes away any toxins or chemicals that do not support your healing process. As you go through a cellular transformation, it is important to drink plenty of water. Some health professionals suggest a litre for every twenty-two kilos of body weight.

There will be times when you may feel disjoined, as though your body is out of phase with everything. This will be frustrating for your mental and emotional bodies. You may feel less functional. This is a natural part of the process as you release the old ways before the new ways can be fully formed. This changeover period may lower your self-esteem sometimes, so it's important to be kind to yourself and relax. It will also bring up a variety of survival issues. You may need to enlist the services of energy healers. Any form of healing acupressure, acupuncture or relaxing massage techniques can help with releasing energies. These energies are held in the crystalline matrix within the structure and tissues of the body. When bodywork is done the connective tissues will start releasing toxins, allowing the healing process to begin. Bodywork such as the aforementioned will help you re-pattern and open your nervous system. It will also break down crystallised energy. Craniosacral therapy and Reiki are also helpful for integrating the energies into your body. There are many homeopathic remedies to try. You may also find that gemstones and Bach flower remedies support your emotional and physical bodies by connecting them to Mother Earth. I often use the combinations found in Sandra Cabot's book *Raw Juices Save Lives*. They have certainly saved me from the stress I experienced ten years earlier when I suffered reflux and constant upper stomach pain. This was diagnosed as a gallbladder stone in my liver partner organ. However, my gut feeling or inner guide told me not to have the gall bladder removal surgery. In desperation and driven by divine guidance, I stumbled upon the juicing book, which featured recipes for most physical discomforts.

How do you break the cycle of emotional energy blocks?

Always speak and think kindly about yourself because your soul needs your love and approval.

As physical lessons have already been learnt, it's now time for our emotional and spiritual sides to be understood so that we can experience what it's like to be whole happy beings. I realise I sometimes still hold emotional grudges, niggles of revenge that are embedded in me at a cellular level. One of my sisters and I could not get along. We somehow radiated the same energy, but with a different purpose. I, not irresponsibly, accused her of being controlling. I told her the whole family was affected and that I felt I had to counteract to help our tamed, battered, soft-hearted siblings. One of our mother's teachings was to always be kind and giving, to surrender during misunderstandings and avoid further conflicts. Well, being born under the sun of Libra, it was very difficult for me not to react when family differences occurred. As a young girl, my reactions were perhaps a threat to my sister. During our younger days there were times when our nice chats suddenly turned into nasty arguments. This made me smile remembering how silly emotions can be at times.

Most conflicts occur when the emotions with negative energy, like jealousy or deep-seated hatred, are present. These controlling behaviours may be inherited from someone along the timeline of our life. Negative energy can only be corrected if the person is aware of the life pattern cycle and exhibits a willingness to change and seek help. The good side of my sister is her generosity, but sometimes this can be a perceived as a disadvantage to the family because it doesn't always seem to be an act of altruism. This may sound judgemental but it's the opinion shared by the rest of the family. My sister's gifts demand reciprocity, which we lowly interpret at times as her being bossy or trying to get her own way. However, someone who is only looking to see the good side in a person might say that this is not really what she is doing; it is actually innocent generosity. This made me realise that our conflicts happened because of my negative reactions. As I was healing my chakras, I started to understand that letting go and surrendering is the key to a peaceful life. Forgiveness is another lesson I learnt from my father. As he was getting older and more vulnerable, things changed. His behaviour radically changed. It was liked things were turned upside down. He became very proud of me, looked up to me and agreed with most of my decisions. His ego dropped and he became almost like my servant. I took it as an apology.

I visited home a few times before he passed on. In that time, my heart slowly opened as I watched him in this very fragile state. He was still tending to his beautiful small garden in the backyard and showed me the fruits of his chilli beans and tomatoes. He was very old, but his green thumb still worked. I was hesitant to go near his garden because of the sad memory still in my heart and mind. Tears appeared in my eyes, for which I had to make excuses so that it was not obvious I was avoiding. All the deep-seated anger and hatred felt was slowly replaced with forgiveness. As I processed this forgiveness in my private place, I felt Mother Mary's energy in me. My eyes poured with tears. The cleansing was occurring. The message to surrender and have peace was now clear. This was something that had previously eluded me because of ego but, as I cleared the layers of my negative beliefs, my life started to become more peaceful and enjoyable. By learning the universe's language, my affirmations and focus are now more suited to my life purpose in living the life of my dreams. There is power in knowing that I am more than enough and I could never comprehend this when I was consumed with illusions of revenge and hatred.

In the case of my relationship with my sister, I used the same process of surrender and forgiveness and chose not to react anymore to her actions. Although we still do not communicate often, our connection as sisters is there and that's all that matters. I enjoy the level of life I'm now in and wish it for everyone, especially to my sister. I am glad that my other siblings have the unlimited patience required to hold the family together. That would have made my mother proud.

Combining all the healing from different healers – spiritual, emotional and physical – I have managed to heal my divine self. I believe everyone deserves to free their lives from the uncomfortable illusion of fear. It is very easy to overcome when you have faith and a connection to your spiritual guides. I can never imagine myself without my guardian angels and my inner guides communicating with each other for my highest good. Without my faith, I would still probably be the same as three quarters of the world's population: killing time from birth to death, as that is all there is for them. By opening my third eye chakra my beautiful mind is now attune with my divine order of life.

It doesn't matter what age you are; life begins at any age. It is never too late, as your soul will continue to journey.

Eight
THE MEDITATION-MINDFUL MEDICINE

'Looking at beauty in the world is the first step of purifying the mind.'

– AMIT RAY

Our brain is made up of billions of brain cells called neurons. These neurons use electricity to communicate with each other and send messages to the whole body. The combination of millions of neurons sending signals at once produces an enormous amount of electrical activity in the brain. This can be detected using sensitive medical equipment, such as an electroencephalogram (EEG), which measures electricity levels over areas of the scalp. The combination of electrical activity of the brain is commonly called a brainwave pattern because of its cyclic wave-like nature. Our mind regulates its activities by means of electrical waves, which are registered by the EEG.

These brainwaves are known as:

- Beta,
- Alpha,
- Theta,
- and Delta.

Beta waves emit when we are consciously alert or feeling agitated, tense or afraid. Their frequencies range from thirteen to sixty pulses per second on the hertz scale, although some science calculates it from fourteen to forty. Beta waves are also associated with alertness, arousal, concentration, cognition and excessive levels of anxiety.

Alpha waves emit when we are in a state of physical and mental relaxation, but remain aware of what is happening around us. Their frequency ranges from seven to thirteen pulses per second. As we close our eyes and become more relaxed, passive or unfocussed, brainwave activity slows down and we produce a burst of alpha wave. When we relax and become mentally unfocussed, alpha waves dominate the brain, producing a calm and pleasant sensation called the alpha state. The alpha state seems to be the brain's neutral or idling state. Healthy people who are under minimal stress tend to produce a lot of alpha activity. Continually lacking alpha activity will follow a sign of anxiety, stress, brain damage, or illness.

Theta wave frequencies are roughly seven pulses per second and cause a state of drowsiness. As calmness and relaxation deepen into drowsiness, the brainwave shifts to slower, more powerfully rhythmic theta waves. Theta has been called the twilight state, as it is between waking and sleeping. It is often accompanied by unexpected dreams or mental images. Often these images are accompanied by vivid memories, particularly childhood memories. Theta offers access to unconscious material, reveries, association, sudden insight and creative ideas. This is the key state in the practice of reality creation.

Delta wave is the state of deep sleep. This frequency emits between one and four cycles per second. During this time, the body enters a state of rejuvenation, recovery and reparation.

In our general waking time, we use the beta brain rhythm. When we start to relax our brain rhythm goes down to alpha. This is the ideal condition for learning new information, such as facts, data or languages. It's also the best time for performing elaborate tasks and analysing complex situations. Meditation or other relaxation exercises are conducive to a sense of calm, which will enable the alpha state.

According to neuroscientists, analysing research participants' electroencephalograms show that being in a state of relaxation causes significant increases in beta levels. It increases endorphins, the neurohormone secreted by the pituitary gland, norepinephrine and dopamine, which is linked to increased mental clarity and memory increase. This effect lasts for hours, sometimes even days, according to Bob Doyle, author of *Wealth Beyond Reason*. This was encouraging to learn, as taking a risk is what led to my present life of peace.

The right hemisphere of the brain is where sympathetic thoughts and creativity originate. It is easy for this hemisphere to create images, make associations, and deal with drawings, diagrams and emotions. The right brain hemisphere is your thinking active mind, and the left side brain hemisphere is your calming side, used for relaxation and healing. Those who have trouble relaxing or sleeping should try blocking their right nostril. Breathing only through your left nostril will help you relax. This technique may even help people suffering from insomnia.

When I meditate on chakra healing I normally use the guided meditation that I created. This is free on my website healingmydivineself.com.au and can be found by clicking the Self-Help tab. With deep breathing, I drift off to theta state. Then, with the guide I trust, my healing mind instructs my body to correct and heal itself.

I remember manifesting a house for my business. I really wanted this house; it was ideal for my intentions and I planned to use it for my new healing business as a sole trader. I viewed this house three times while it was on the market. I memorised every room, from the bedrooms to the dining room, and knew this was the house I wanted. My financial adviser said it was too expensive for me and that I would not be able to afford the monthly payment. He tried negotiating the price down as a favour to me. When his negotiation failed, he told me to leave it, saying it wasn't meant to be. However, my inner guide told me this was the one and I felt that it was really mine. I asked him again to consult the agent one more time. My investment capacity was a maximum of $335,000. If I exceeded that, he calculated that there would be no point, that I would not be able to afford the monthly payment.

The whole afternoon my mind was working something silly. Even when cooking dinner for my daughter I was still focussed on the house. When I went to bed that night, I meditated. I visualised every room, how I would arrange the furniture, how I would turn the big unneeded dining room into five bedrooms. The front room would be used as a lounge room, which would be ideal for my clinic. I drifted away, my brainwave now indicating I was in the theta state. I continued to visualise until I fell asleep. The next day my financial adviser rang me. He said he didn't know what happened but the real estate agent rang him at nine in the morning to tell him the owner was now willing to sell it for $335,000!

I started to advertise the place for boarders. I only needed one room for my clinic so the rest could be rented out. This was my original plan if I ever bought this house. I was still working at the casino as a croupier, which proved ideal as I was able to advertise the rooms for rent there by word of mouth. The transition was pleasant as it was divinely guided. At five years old I'd had dreams of owning big houses. Somehow they kept happening and I was always very grateful. This house has also proven beneficial, especially for my clients who require accessibility. My ex-mother-in-law was still very active at that time and used to come to visit. She stayed with us on school holidays when she was still able to drive and even offered to stay with my daughter while I was busily working two jobs. At that time, I was still taking four to five clients out of madness and excitement every afternoon. I was able to keep this routine going for a while and am very grateful to my mother-in-law, who used to get upset whenever I introduced her as my *ex*-mother-in-law! She said she did not divorce me; her son did. I felt honoured. We got along very well. She sometimes stays at our place for weeks with her spoilt white dog that has slowly learned to get along with my cheeky puppies.

On my day off from the casino I had eight clients, four of whom had knee problems. Since last week, one had ridden her bike – something she hadn't done for years due to her bad knee. She was trying to prove to me that she'd gotten better after just one treatment. Signs of trust and faith like this made me even more grateful. This client can now bend her knee again and do her gardening. She has since come back for another treatment.

It was a long and productive day. When I got home my mother-in-law already had dinner ready. My daughter and I always felt spoiled when she was around. After dinner, I retired before them to ensure I got enough rest for my four-am start at the casino. I thanked them both for the day and they decided to stay up late watching movies. I did not mind, it being a school holiday, and they always enjoy each other's company. Lying in bed feeling grateful for my day, I slowly wound my brain down. I was feeling sleepy and my mind wandered to thinking about how it would feel to have a sore knee. As I mentioned in the last chapter, be careful with your thoughts as they can manifest. My alarm went off at three in the morning as normal. My routine is: no mucking around, get up, get ready and go off to work. Well, this particular morning was different. I could not get up. Both of my knees were in so much pain that I had to hold on to the walls to go to the bathroom. Oh dear. I couldn't recall any obvious incident that would've damaged my knees this way. All I could remember was wondering how it would feel to have a sore knee before falling asleep. I must have manifested this thought while in my meditative state on the theta brainwave. I had to make a phone call to my shift manager, informing them that I would not be able to come to work. My knee was in pain for a week. At that time, I was not yet practising my energy healing work nor was I aware of my energy healing gift. These days, I can shift this kind of acute discomfort in five minutes. My managers were concerned because I never took sick days. My record in my last appraisal was no sick leave for five years unless I went to a seminar. At all times, the scheduling department were very supportive, for which I was grateful.

The high heel-induced neck pain I mentioned in the last chapter was my starting point for learning how to integrate energy healing with meditation. Being unable to move the entire left side of my body, I was left to be still and meditate. Here I was, setting my intentions to rid myself of the pain I did not want to own. It was horrible. My beta waves as usual were running a thousand miles a minute. I was just the same as seventy-five percent of the population. I had no idea how to quieten my mind, so concentrated as my inner-self guide says, counting my breaths, holding for a few counts at the top of an inhalation then exhaling before repeating. Eventually my body continued this involuntarily until I managed to hold my breath for longer than twelve counts. A few years later I found out that this technique is called the Buteyko method of breathing. It is an alternative breathing technique to help the body correct a lot of illnesses that medications do not affect. Also having the intention to heal makes it easier for your body to follow your mind's instructions.

As you go down to alpha waves make sure to focus on your intention. Beta waves will still pop up sometimes, so try to change your effort to match your purpose. It's critical to maintain your focus as your brainwaves drip down to theta wave. This is where manifestations occur just before going to delta wave and indicates that your body is now gearing up to repair and rejuvenate while manifesting your other desires.

Meditation practice can be done anywhere. All you need to do is be mindful, have good thoughts and focus on your breathing. I would suggest to always be mindful, as you never know what your subconscious will take on board. The meditation I did for the manifestation of my house was what an expert called a 'reflective meditation', which is thinking about a specific subject or theme. It is the simplest form of meditation and is well-suited for beginners.

Many eastern approaches, like those practised by monks, involve using a passive style of meditation. This is where empty your mind through relaxation until you can observe your own thoughts as if you are somehow separate from them. It's like watching a movie about yourself. Passive meditation should ideally be practised fifteen to twenty minutes daily, preferably first thing in the morning. However, three times a week would also suffice for those with busier lifestyles. Alternatively, you can practise a smaller variation during your breaks at work and then do a proper one when you return home. This practice reduces stress, improves concentration and encourages creativity and inspiration.

Here are a few guidelines on how to meditate.

Sit comfortably in a chair with a good back support either in a quiet room or in a garden. I prefer to sit in the garden with my feet planted comfortably on the ground to centre myself. I place my hands on my lap with my palms facing up if I am asking to receive something from the divine source, and facing down when I am sending healing energy to someone far away.

When you're all set, close your eyes. Empty your lungs and breathe in deeply through your nose. Do not strain. Simply become aware of your breath as it flows in and out.

For grounding, concentrate on your feet and let go. Relax them and thank the universe for this opportunity. Slowly draw the energy from the Mother Earth and guide it so that it comes up through your legs, upper body and head. Now imagine the orbs of the golden healing light from the divine source pouring down over your head. Feel that divine energy healing your whole body, checking every part of it, making sure every cell is repairing and rejuvenating. You will feel a tingle down your spine as the cerebral fluids trickle down with good healthy trace elements to the rest part of your body. Using meditation techniques gave me the spiritual support to heal my divine self.

Nine

LIFE PURPOSE – HEAL FOR PURPOSE

'The meaning of life is to find your gift and the purpose of life is to give it away.'

– **Anonymous**

My challenges were part of my divine order of life. It took me a long time to understand and discover this. Although I was a slow learner, the path of my past experiences kept interrupting my direction until I learned to let go and focus only on what I desire. Life in the Philippines – especially village existence – was not without its difficulties and survival was the main modus operandi for most. During discussions with my relatives on visits to my village, I was told that my mother borrowed money from her friends to buy food whenever we had guests. This could have been our relatives on my father's side visiting from far away or just random friends chilling out at our farmhouse. My mother and her family always treated people with pure love and innocence, as this was an accepted part of village life. Unfortunately the culture changed when rebels – mainly gangs of criminals and radicals who opposed the government – forced this way of life to near extinction. Trust and friendship faded from our village and corruption became a way of life.

When my brother was accepted to join the army my mother had mixed emotions. I could imagine her feelings vacillating between pride, anxiousness and worry every time my brother came home for visits. The rebel forces in our area were known to attack families who had close connections with the government and my brother, being in the army, fitted this description. I noticed there was always a tinge of sadness on my mother's face, even when she was happy. At this time, I started to read people's feelings from the pattern of their expressions. I think I inherited this trait from my mum, but I lost it when I adopted a different lifestyle in the big city. Alcohol fogged up my mind and took over, boosting my ego. The money I had created an imbalance within me that I could not figure out. I felt ashamed having so much money, as I never had it when I was back at the farm. It felt unfair to others who worked so hard for little just to meet their needs.

The blockage was in my receiving chakra. Instead of going with the flow I sabotaged by giving away money to undeserving people who would use it to gamble or buy alcohol. This abundance of money and my ego drew me to reality. I questioned why money was not always earned in a meaningful way.

Since I have started healing my chakras, the shame of receiving has dissipated. I understand the law of vibration and attraction: what I project towards the universe is what I get back tenfold. My relationship to everything and everyone has started to make sense. In Australia, I am fortunate to own a car to drive to work and back and to do my shopping within a ten-kilometre distance. I noted that most vehicles were similar and it was just normal owning an unreliable vehicle when we are in our limiting beliefs. We do not notice a difference in the quality of life we are in. We become used to life in suburbia. In the environment I lived in the cycle or pattern of existence was to spend weekends partying and consuming too much alcohol. This was so different to my life at home on the farm back in the Philippines. Many times business deals or opportunities turned out to be totally disingenuous – sometimes even illegal. You sort yourself out, stress and anxiety prevailing, and the so-called caring friends leave, retreating to their own safety. Some people are stuck in the ruts but don't realise it. I was just naïve and didn't know that I could create a dream life. I used to please friends and join in even though I did not really like what they were doing. I wished to be someone else; I was in hiding and not my authentic self at all. When I was invited to a party it took two hours for me to get ready because none of the clothes in my wardrobe looked nice on me. I used to criticise myself. I was my own worst enemy for a long time until I learned to tap into my inner guides and divine source from loving spirits and angels.

My body's aches and pain are spiritual messages that help me find my way back to who I am and what am I here to be. Negative emotions contributed to all my physical discomforts. They also helped me understand the process of letting go and surrendering, something I could never do thirty years ago. At that time I considered giving up a defeat. My ego-driven mind convinced me to hold on to my negative beliefs. I was not even aware of it; it was operating at a subconscious or DNA level.

Nowadays I have changed the choice of my words. I try to be positive and watch my thoughts all the time because I now love and respect myself. Whenever I stuff up I forgive myself and keep going. Stress is no longer an issue. When I see clients, I can straightaway pick up the negative habits that are contributing to their imbalances, whether spiritual, emotional or physical.

A few weeks after moving in, one of my roomers found her working hours drastically reduced and was unable to pay her rent for four weeks. I noted the conversation she had with me every time I asked how her day was. The stories she shared were predominantly about others' negative behaviours – whether it was her ex-husband, friends or her bosses. She even started noticing the changes and weaknesses of other roomers in the house, which was not a problem to me before she had moved in. This sweet-looking girl's choices and the way she thought about and saw every person in a negative light actually changed the energy around my environment. Dense energy started to emerge and things became unpleasant. Her struggle to retain jobs affected me slightly as she was not able to pay rent anymore for awhile. It would've been easy said and done to kick her out, but my divine self did not agree with this idea. One night I visualised her handing me her rent money during my meditation and, the next morning, she called to tell me she'd gotten paid and had already put money into my account.

The crux of my workshop presentation teaches you to clear unwanted energy and replace it with what you desire. The life purpose I am unwittingly following is now leading me to help people to live better. I ultimately want to assist people so that they see the big picture opening up. I want them to unpack their own gifts and potential. During sessions, I ask my client to choose an oracle card. This guides me to elaborate, as guided by the angels and other loving spirits, when my clients are not yet ready to understand the meaning or clue within their card's messages. In the process of clearing blocks and healing your divine self, your mind will, in its own time, open up to your desires and you will start working on getting there.

Ten

BONUSES – DIVINE SELF HEALING TIPS

Let's start cleansing your chakras. It is important to check in with our chakras on a daily basis to live our lives to the fullest. Here is how you can energise your chakras:

- Take salt baths. For thousands of years sea salt baths were a common way to relax your whole body. Himalayan salt is the best. They cleanse the body's energy system, allowing the energy centres to clearly express. Visualising your energy centre makes it more powerful as the clearing of your chakras will revitalise you at the same time.

- Bless your food. Take a moment to pray and say thanks to the universe for the food that you are about to consume. Food helps you maintain your vitality, so bless it with love to open up your energy centres (chakras). I occasionally eat meat; however, in my prayer I focus on the animals that were sacrificed for my food and ask the angels to help them get to a comfortable place that has an abundance of what they need.

- You can also do some exercise to exert excess energy and calm your mind. I enjoy walking my dog for two hours. While mindfully walking, good ideas come to me and I ask my guardian angels to help me retain these ideas until I get home to write it down. Seeing beautiful gardens around my neighbourhood makes my energy vibration feel higher. Maintaining beautiful thoughts and holding up good feelings attracts and invites good things to come into my life. Feeling good is a sign that your chakras are alive and filled with vital force.

Food choice is important. You should eat foods that your body can easily recognise. I always have all-year-round greens in my garden and herbs like **lemon grass**, which is purifying, stimulating and refreshing for the mind. This is helpful for mental fatigue and loss of connection and is an excellent tonic when recovering from illness as it stimulates glandular secretion and the digestive process. It encourages appetite and may help with gastric problems.

Citrus plants, like limes, lemons, and mandarins, are also very useful. Not only can you use them for marinating or cooking, but you can also use the young leaves or skin for a breathing exercise. Soak the plant it in a hot water bowl and breathe through your nostrils. Cover your head with a towel and stick close to the bowl so that you can inhale and absorb the scented steam. This is helpful for uplifting and is useful for listlessness, depression, anxiety and nervousness. It also encourages restful sleep and helps instil confidence. It is also valuable as an intestinal antiseptic and can relieve conditions such as painful indigestion. I use **bergamot essential oil**, the extract oil form of citrus plant flowers, during massage or with an oil burner to promote good sleep.

Cinnamon is one ingredient I cannot run out in my herbs cupboard. I mix this with my organic coffee most mornings, as this is known to lower blood pressure. It is also good for easing mental fatigue, tension, treating depression and diminishing life's pressure. This can also be purchased in essential oil form. Cinnamon and chilli powder coffee is my favourite drink in the morning. Have you ever tried chilli coffee? **Chillies** actually help stimulate your brain. Their heat comes from capsaicin, which is found in the seeds, white membranes and the flesh. According to Dr Sandra Cabot, capsaicin can block the activation of cancer-causing chemicals and encourages the release of endorphins – chemicals in the brain which improve mood and circulation, relieve sinus and catarrh, and assist with weight loss by increasing the metabolic rate. Be cautioned that you might not be able to consume this if you have a sensitive digestive system or intestinal problems.

Spinach and silverbeet are all over my back garden. These heal and help the lining of the digestive tract. They also improve vision and can reduce arthritic pain. This is thanks to two key nutrients:

- Choline, an essential micronutrient helps with the metabolisation of fatty acids in the liver, and

- Inositol, a vital cofactor for the brain's major neurotransmitters.

Inositol is essential for brain and nervous system health. It is also good for maintaining healthy blood vessels and supports kidney and liver function. This is especially helpful for anaemia sufferers. It can also reduce heavy menstrual bleeding and reduces fatigue and constipation.

Tomatoes and **capsicums** are good for the heart. They also support the liver by cleansing its bile. They have antiseptic properties to help reduce infections and are helpful for high blood pressure, gout and kidney/bladder problems. It is, however, advisable to consume these in moderation as over-indulging in these can sometimes cause reflux.

There are some vegetables that I do not have in my garden all year round. I try to find these in organic vegetable markets, ensuring they are as free of pesticides as possible. Fresh food is ultimately all you need to support optimal body function.

Additional Tips for Signature Food:

- Walnuts and cauliflowers are a good support food for your brain – they even look like brains, don't they? These are familiar vegetables for everyone in the vegetable market.

- Carrots and kiwi fruits offer very good support for your eyes. Next time you cut a carrot, take a good look and notice it looks like the pupils of your eyes.

- Mushrooms are a good support for your thyroid. A sliced mushroom looks a lot like your thyroid, and will miraculously help to restore that organ. Like blueberries, mushrooms can heal your throat chakra.

- Grapes a great support for your gall bladder. They also help combat anaemia and blood disorders and provide a quick boost of physical energy. Grapes can reduce the inflammation of arthritis and eliminate acids from the body to improve complexions. They have a laxative effect and diuretic properties.

- Broccoli is a signature food for lungs, but is also excellent for weight loss and for treating high blood pressure, liver problems and constipation.

Supporting Your Lungs

A friendly note to all smokers: it is important to support your lungs just like your other organs. Don Tolman, author of *Farmacist Desk Reference*, noted that our lungs are made up of hundreds of thousands of branching tubes that end in tiny air sacs or alveoli. There are over 300 million of these tiny sacs in our lungs, offering roughly the surface area of a tennis court to keep up with the respiratory demands of the body. The membranes of these tiny air sacs are also thinner than tissue paper to maximise the exchange of gasses. Our lungs make up a large part of our immune system. Pollutants and infections that cause microbes are captured by mucus in the lungs and shuttled upward by a tiny brass-like organelle that is known in medical terms as cilia. This causes us to cough or swallow. Sneezes are another way the lungs rid themselves of infection or pollution before the invaders pass beyond our sinuses.

The lungs are a remarkable pair of organs that should be cared for. Smoking is the most damaging habit for this organ as it destroys cilia, which prevent the clogging of the airways. Our body needs good amount of oxygen to burn fuel, such as sugars and fatty food, and turn them into energy. Healthy lungs are important as they help us breathe in air, the vital life force for cells and other organs. A well-hydrated body with an abundance of oxygen is less likely to contract diseases like cancer as cancer cell cannot live in a well-hydrated oxygenated body. Your best bet is to maintain a healthy diet with minimal sugar.

Supporting Your Heart

Capsicums and tomatoes should be a staple part of your diet and it's a good idea to start your day with a steaming bowl of oats. These are full of omega-3 fatty acids, foliate and potassium. This fibre-rich food can help lower cholesterol and keep arteries clear.

Supporting Your Uterus

Avocados are a good support for the uterus. Note that it takes nine months for an avocado to progress from flowering to maturation – exactly the same as the gestation period for a foetus in a mother's womb. Combine them with alfalfa and other bean sprouts, which are good for maintaining reasonable counts of oestrogen, to support women through menopausal transition. At the age of forty-seven I started to experienced high blood pressure. I was taking Micardis, a receptor blocker, to help lower it, but it caused me to develop a dry cough. My blood pressure was successfully lowered, but even after a foot reflexology treatment the cough persisted. I went back to my general practitioner for a blood test to investigate my declining health.

After three days my doctor called and said the result had come back. He needed to see me personally, as what he had to say could not be discussed over the phone. Naturally, I started to have concerns. I did not wait another day to find out; I had to go and see my doctor straight away. He explained to me that my oestrogen count was only 100, while a normal count was at least 600. He asked if I wanted him to prescribe me a hormone replacement, but I refused, saying that I would work on it and return in three months for another checkup. After a crazy three months of juicing, meditation, exercise and eating alfalfa bean sprouts and other super fresh vegetables, my oestrogen count increased to 400. I also stopped taking the high blood pressure tablets and felt my energy levels improving. By adopting a new lifestyle and changing my diet I made a huge difference both mine and my family's quality of life.

Supporting Your Kidneys and Bones

Including more beans in your diet, like broad beans, is a great way to support your kidneys.

The best food for your strong bones is celery. It's no coincidence that it looks just like your femur or thighbone! It is also beneficial for treating arthritis, gout and toxicity. Because it is a natural diuretic it is excellent for treating stomach acidity and reflux. It can reduce fluid retention, calm the nervous system, help balance the body's PH level and can be helpful for insomnia sufferers and those with kidney issues, bladder problems or even constipation.

Here are more specific food types that, as recorded in many health journals, can help as a male enhancer.

- Chilli peppers contain potassium, which improves heart health and circulation, leading to increased sexual stamina. In addition, chilli peppers have been shown to reduce inflammation, improve digestive health and boost immunity.

- Whole grains and beans are rich in thiamine, a B vitamin that stimulates the nervous system. The nervous system plays an important role in sexual performance, as it allows you to interpret signals and feelings. Enhanced sensitivity means performance will typically last longer. Whole grains and beans are also good for heart health, the digestive system and are important for maintaining muscles mass and increasing all-around physical strength.

- Acerola cherries are the best source of vitamin C. They are thirteen times better than orange juice. This important micronutrient improves blood flow throughout the body and boosts the immune system. Additionally, acerola are a great source of anthocyanins, a subclass of flavonoids that enhance blood flow. Flavonoids also act as an antioxidant, slow the ageing process and fight chronic disease by reducing damage to cells and DNA.

- Flaxseeds are a rich source of omega fatty acids, which are important for maintaining blood flow to the sexual organs and throughout the rest of the body. Omega-3 is important in formation of the male sex hormone testosterone, the production of which declines as men get older or suffer chronic stress.

- Bananas have many benefits when it comes to natural male enhancement. They are a great source of potassium that helps balance out excess sodium in the body, improving heart health and increasing stamina. Bananas are also a source of vitamin B6, which is believed to help stimulate the growth of penis tissue. Aside from sexual heath benefits, bananas are great for general health. They contain a wide range of important vitamins and minerals as well as dietary, fibre and antioxidants.

- Nuts, such as walnuts, Brazil nuts and pecans, are a great source of omega-3 fatty acids. Consuming nuts enhances blood flow to the sexual organs and help in the production of testosterone. They are high in amino acids, which help reduce impotency and improve the quality of erections. They are also known to improve brain health and help maintain cognitive function.

- Garlic. Garlic contains a concentration of the compound allicin, which has been shown to increase blood flow to the genital region. This allows for stronger and longer-lasting erections. Garlic also helps to cut cholesterol levels, clearing the arteries and reducing the risk of coronary heart disease.

- Dark chocolate (seventy to ninety percent cocoa) should be consumed in moderation, but is also a food for the third eye chakra. It contains substantial amounts of the chemical serotonin, which can enhance the sensitivity of the nervous system and promote the release of feel-good hormones from the brain. This can increase sexual desire and enhance feelings of pleasure. Dark chocolate also lowers the risk of heart disease and contains antioxidants that can help to slow the ageing process.

The vegetables listed in the chakra chapter are a small starting point. It is now up to your imagination to broaden your tastes and resources in your pursuit of excellent health. Food is nature's medicine. In one of his seminars, Don Tolman quoted Hippocrates, saying 'Let thy food be thy medicine and medicine be thy food.' Our bodies are composed of millions of tubes and if some of them become blocked we get into trouble. If you eat foods that are covered with chemicals and preservatives your body will have trouble digesting them, which will cause a blockage in your system. Yuck!

Since my daughter's episode twenty-five years ago I am mindful of every medication we take. I learned to listen to the parts of my body that were giving me discomfort, as this was a sign that something wasn't right in my energy channel. If you have been following my advice since the angel light in chapter four, you should already be in tune and connected with your body and angel guides. For example, I experienced lower abdominal pains and, being in tune with my energy channel, I was told to heat up a wheat bag and place it on top of my ankles. Being familiar with body reflex points, I knew that ankles are actually a gynaecological reflex point. After five minutes of restful application, my lower abdomen pain banished. I noted these little messages when I studied chakra healing. They made sense. My base chakra could also need cleansing and activating.

Another time I was called to do a distant healing by someone who could not come to my clinic. A friend's son had a facial reconstruction after a cricket accident and needed something to relax him and help him get some sleep. The boy's father, who I used to connect with, held his son's hand while I performed the distant healing. His hand started heating up and slowly his son relaxed and fell asleep.

When we finished the session, I developed headaches so I drank water to hydrate my brain. Normally this makes me feel better, but this time the pain increased. It was one o'clock on a thirty-degree summer's day. My angel guide told me to go out into the sun, but I did not. My ego-driven mind prevented me because it knew that sun is ordinarily not good if you have a migraine or headache. As most migraine sufferers can attest, it actually triggers those discomforts. All I could do was lie in bed with this pounding headache, sipping water every few minutes and ignoring the divine message. The message kept nudging me to go out in the sun. It was already five o'clock and the trees in my backyard were shadowing the sun. My pain was getting worse, so I finally gave in and thought, okay, nothing to lose. I found a spot to sit where there was just a little sun left to shine on me. I closed my eyes and felt the warmth of what little sun was left. Two minutes after my head felt lighter. I could feel something lift off out of my fontanelle, the top of my head where my crown chakra was.

Concentration had depleted my crown chakra energy and I had just needed to get my balance back. When I was younger, I would take aspirin or painkillers straight away, but now I know that medication or food that has plenty of preservatives can also clog your tubes.

Eleven

ABUNDANCE/FINANCES THE UNLIMITED SOURCE

'Abundance is not something we acquire; it is something we turn into.'
–Wayne Dyer

Have you heard stories from people who work very hard their whole lives, but say they are always broke? Or as soon as they save up, another bill becomes due and they are back to nothing. Sound familiar? I used to feel that way, too.

Some people on pension benefits choose to work only a few hours a week because they fear that earning more will alter or even deny them their pension allowance. Another classic belief: when you earn more you are taxed more.

These are limiting beliefs. When we send them out into the universe, we get double in return until we change our view and perception… Cycles of poverty occur because the mind has been set to those beliefs. People either set these themselves or they are set by parents or a past generation. These cycles become a reality, blocking abundance in their lives. I once heard my ex-husband's friend say, 'Blessings are not shared fairly and equally' and he is one of the less beneficial ones. It's not your fault if you have inherited a limiting belief, but you don't have to continue the trend. Hopefully this chapter will open up your blocked channel so that you can recreate your life to be prosperous just by changing your mindset. You can empower yourself by focussing on happiness and gratitude. Be happy to wake up every morning. The sun is shining and the rain just right for the gardens. Remember a happy memory, like the love and joy you felt when your child was born. Be grateful to share meals with family and friends and enjoy the good health that comes from choosing the right foods and preparing them correctly. If you do this and maintain a positive outlook your financial needs will be met.

You'll be able to replace your worries and stress with trust and faith.

The whole universe is breathing like we are. The chakra energy within your being is your connection, your antennae to catch the universe's vibrations, which radiate every second. It may not know the specifics, but it is always there to respond to your energy vibration frequency. But if you are not aware of all this, how can you make a change?

I am very grateful to my spiritual guide for pointing me towards forensic energy healing. With this, I managed to recognise the layers of negative blocks in my energy field which were preventing me from moving forward and fully accepting who I was and what I was here to be. Achieving is feeling the outcome of what you have desired and feeling excited that you already have it. Train your mind and heart to feel this and allow your situation to alter your life without you controlling the process. Challenges might be temporarily experienced during the process, but keep in mind that there is always calm after the storm. This is how the universe helps you achieve your goals. Learn to go with the flow as it's important to find balance for your new mindset. The key is to have patience and be kind to yourself. The disasters that are happening around the world (i.e. earthquakes, typhoons, tornados, floods) are happening because the Mother Earth is stressed. She is trying to restore balance, while we humans continue to destroy. It's not worth it to stress and worry, as this will only bring about more of the same. I understand some people find it difficult to alter ingrained habits. I was the same until I had the forensic healing sessions, which helped me remember and return to who I once was and erase all the negative beliefs I'd inherited as they were not serving my purpose. Acknowledging the presence and assistance of angels certainly helps us. They are always ready to take on anything we share with them, and wait for us to acknowledge and invite them to guide us. Surrender and let them take your stress and worries from you, and slowly watch your life change. I always ask them to guide my words, actions and thoughts so that they are always in alignment with my desires. That way I am always guided to only think positively and, when I speak, the words I use can be helpful for everyone.

My intention is to be free from limiting beliefs. I feel this from my solar plexus, my third or 'power' chakra. It causes me to experience a nice tingly feeling that connects to my heart chakra. The heart is a regulator that aligns other chakras to the divine source and Mother Earth. With your powerful mind, they will work together to deliver that feeling to the whole body. When you communicate with your inner guides make sure to use the words that they can understand so they can serve your purpose. Let me try this dialogue with you. For example, you would like to take your family on a holiday next year on December 21. You must have a specific date in mind to make it a more genuine promise. That way you can really hold yourself accountable for it. You can say, 'What would it take for me to bring my family on a very nice holiday?' The next thing is to imagine your holiday destination, wherever that may be. Imagine the activities you will do everyday with your family, feel the joy and excitement, the taste of the local food you will be trying for the first time, the room that you chose with the massive window and nice view. Let your imagination run wild. It will raise your vibration to the level of the angels and help realise your dreams. Follow your intuition and do whatever is necessary. It could be some overtime work to earn extra cash. Keep following your plan through.

When you tap in to spirituality, you must focus on what you desire. Your determination to fulfil your desires will then be supported by money that will suddenly come from different sources. To manifest financial abundance, you must have a reason for why you need money. It is better to visualise your figure and purpose. Just remember that money is an energy to help you evolve easily. All my manifestations happened by following those simple instructions with my inner self. I own oracle cards by Doreen Vertue. Every now and then I pick a card to receive messages from the angels. I thought about how my financial situation needs some improvement and picked a card. It said to concentrate on my service. My understanding here was that if you concentrate, work to the best of your ability and make your boss happy, you might get a promotion and increase your earnings.

Our spiritual guides and angels have ways of helping us. I remember one experience that I cannot forget. My daughter hosted a party to help a friend who was starting a party planning business. My daughter's job as host was to sell as many goods as possible. This would get her more free items for herself. I, of course, wanted to help, as all mothers do. I ended up ordering $500 worth of stuff – which was more than I could afford. I realised this after the party, so asked Archangel Michael to help me obtain enough money to pay for my order before it arrived in two weeks. My ego mind told me to buy a lottery ticket and hope to win enough for my order. The next day I eagerly checked the results to see if some of my numbers had come up. Better luck next time. Not to worry. I never get disappointed. I followed through the guide that I now understand from my ego. I was overwhelmed trying to find ways to make money and was not listening properly. I acted without communicating with my spiritual guides. After three days, I received mail from the bank out of the blue. It was a notification that I had accumulated points by using my credit card.

The points equated to $500, which was automatically deposited into my savings account following an easy internet banking process.

Archangel Michael also helped me with my electricity bills. I paying more than a thousand dollars every quarter due to the few roomers I had in the house. One day I asked to have my bills taken care of, as they were way too high – even after a solar electricity system was installed. To my surprise, my electricity provider sent me a letter informing me that they'd made a mistake and were overcharging me. They apologised and explained that the next power bill would be covered, as my account was in credit. I had even accumulated credit from the bills I had already paid over the whole year.

Time Abundance

For awhile, my time was very limited, as I was working two jobs. I asked the universe, divine source, angels what it would take to gain more time for myself and for the people I loved: my family and friends.

I really enjoyed my job at the casino and was grateful for it. The interactions I had with my co-staff members, bosses and customers were always pleasant. I didn't even mind the 4 am starts. I still enjoyed it and always looked forward to travelling from one job to the other. After my divine request for more time, the energy at the casino started to change. I suddenly feeling I should not be there anymore. Structural and conceptual improvements to the building were starting to stress most of the employees out and the mangers expected us to meet their demands in a shorter timeframe. Everyone was forced to step out of their comfort zone. Remember: calmness allows follows the storm, so chaos has to be experienced. A new system was introduced and everyone in the gaming department had to re-learn their roles. This prepared me to take on my request, which I did not understand at that time. But then one of my bosses tried to operate in ways that put the company's interests above its employees. She was following her own strong beliefs. Her approach was not pleasant to some employees – mostly to women – and I was not expecting to share their experience, being an easygoing flexible person. However, it soon became my time to be picked on. It was a very unpleasant experience that changed my day-to-day balance. I was not feeling excited to go to work anymore. I was making silly mistakes in a job I had done for almost thirty years. Her continued harassment drew me to finally request a confrontational meeting with the human resources management to resolve the issue of her negative accusations. Normality and my enjoyment of the job only returned when she was absent from the workplace.

It was not a nice experience for either of us, but it had to be brought out into the open so that fairness in the workplace would prevail. Reviewing their practices was already overdue, as they were hoping to bring the casino in line with their advertising and make it a better place to work with a friendly atmosphere. When asking for intervention from the divine source, remember that the process will not always be the icing of the cake of life. I was still very grateful for the outcome. I was no longer in two minds about quitting. The money I earned from the job was no longer meaningful. Instead of adding it to my investment I could not wait to spend this toxic money. Quitting my job was a part of my blessings; I could enjoy time with my family and grandson anytime of the day. The clients I attracted through my healing work were grateful for the improved availability of my service, which left me feeling rewarded everyday of my life. I did not understand it at first until I started enjoying my life with my purpose. I managed my time without any pressure. It was pleasant and time was always available to do the things I enjoyed most.

Twelve

THE NEXT GENERATION

'Treat a child as though he already is a person he's capable of becoming.'
– HAIM GINOTT

My mother was the most influential person in my life. Her wisdom, love and the compassion that she possessed continually operate behind my subconscious, keeping me inspired in my day-to-day adventure. Life, to me, is an adventure. My partner and I often talk about generations, the economy, the way everything evolves. He is scientifically minded, while I am more into spirituality. He often talks about the economy and the politicians, a topic that normally stresses people who watch the news out. For that reason, I cut down on listening to the news on television and the media in general. After a few exchanged words, I was told I could not bury my face in the sand all the time. My reactions to that comment sometimes challenge my peaceful mind and can almost lead to an argument. Thankfully I admire my partner in other ways. He has the ability to cool off the conversation and make it humorous, rather than allowing it to become a real debate. I understood he was fearful about the future of the economy. 'If we do not do the right thing, what will happen to the future generation?' he says.

A desire to control is a sign of fear. If we cannot let go of the things that are beyond our control, we will slowly introduce stress into our lives. Sometimes this cannot be helped when, like my partner, we care so much.

We all have fear. This protector emotion prevents us from hurting ourselves, but it can also be a negative force stopping us from moving forward. If you are an achiever you would probably call this form of fear 'stress'.

Stress is FEAR (False Evidence Appearing Real). We all experience it in some context during our lives. It could be fear of rejection, fear of failure, fear of being alone, fear of success, fear of love, or fear of the unknown. These emotions have been hardwired into all human beings for generations and we continue to pass them down without even knowing it.

How do we break this cycle to our next generations? By guiding our children and showing them how to be empowered and responsible for their own actions. They must be taught how to love, respect and appreciate others. I trust these three foundations most, as they will truly make a difference. Parents are role models and children will follow everything they do. Most parents tell their kids 'no' to almost everything at a very young age when they are exploring. Yes, raising and balancing a powerful individual is a full responsibility. Children are individuals with their own personalities and adults need to grow and adjust with them. Parenting is a skill that I really enjoy. Although I've only had one parenting experience, I came from a big family so I understand the way our mother guided and grew with each of us. Parents may lay a good foundation by showing children what they want them to become. This takes time and parents are often too busy nowadays to spend a lot of quality time with their kids. They need to go to work to keep up the standard they have set for their children's future. The children are their future, their main investments, and need to be focussed on above all else. Your views may differ. I was fortunate to have my mother-in-law assisting us at all times during the early days of parenting our child. We had the same bond beliefs and taught my daughter the difference between right and wrong. That was all we needed.

After clearing the negative blockages caused by my childhood experiences, I learnt a valuable lesson about how to raise my child. My mother's method of disciplining was to let us kneel for a length of time based on the severity of our naughtiness. I found it effective for us. We became more responsible at an early age doing allocated chores that varied according to our capabilities. These ranged from gathering chickens to their nest for the night so they didn't sleep all over the yard to feeding pigs and buffalos. All of these jobs were shared and it was my older brother's responsibility to make sure we were doing them correctly. Being in charged, he was allowed to reprimand us when things were not done properly.

The discussion my partner and I had about the economy is different, as my attitude now is based on spirituality, purpose and the belief that I am more than enough. The power of every word guides me towards the feeling of contentment and the universe reacts towards the vibrations I am radiating. I am no longer eager to horde money in preparation for future crises. This fear of future crises makes people feel sick. It has already caused weakened and stressed kidneys. I no longer worry about yesterday and tomorrow, as these two days do not apply in spiritual life. The closer they interact with this energy the more vulnerable a person will be to negativity, greed, or even crimes, creating disaster unto oneself. One person sending energy out can affect 227 people. Imagine that! This has been calibrated by energy experts. Energy will always affect people, regardless of whether it is positive or negative. The choice is plain and easy: what kind of energy do we want to radiate if we want to create a better world?

The challenges we face everyday are our teachers in the school of life. We must understand that physical and emotional pains, and even financial troubles, are just reminders that we are derailing ourselves from the life we are meant to have.

I watch my pets expressing their happiness and serenity, feeling content as their authentic selves, as I radiate positive energy towards them. To me, this is evidence of my positive evolution.

On the other hand, seeing young children with erratic personalities makes you wonder what kind of energy their raisers are projecting towards them. It may seem obvious and it is easy to judge the way these parents and children operate. It might seem wrong to ethical people, but it's all they know. They believe they are doing their best. Instead of judging and criticising, we can actually take this as a blessing and make a change for ourselves. We should radiate positive energy, showing love to ourselves and others. Be thoughtful and kind to all creatures and other earth walkers, as the universe reacts to positive emotions. Slowly you will notice positive changes in your surroundings. This becomes your new world. Remember the 227 individuals that you are affected by? The positive energy you direct towards each of them will continue to radiate the same. With the hope of change we can then commence evolution.

The other day I went with my daughter and fourteen-month-old grandson to a new play centre. This play centre was fully equipped with facilities for children of all ages, and the coffee bar was magnificent. It was perfect for my daughter as it gave her the opportunity to have a break and enjoy morning tea in peace. I volunteered to watch my grandson while playing on the baby section play pen with other babies. At this stage, he was going through a biting phase, so I was instructed to keep one eye on the little biter. As predicted, he very quickly tried to grab and bite the other young ones as soon as he got close. My daughter's fear of taking him out on her own was understandable, especially given she was six months pregnant with her second child. A few minutes later new young ones came along. I intended to let my grandson stay so that he would get used to other babies his age. I was bitten once as I covered his mouth to stop him biting. One mother said it was okay to let him be close to her baby; she had no idea how painful my hand was from the bite I'd received a few minutes earlier.

I followed my grandson closely, keeping an eye on him. I thought if I let him get used to other children for awhile it might break his bad habit and improve his social skills. It's important to understand that the brains of children aged one to seven are like sponges absorbing what they observe. They are innocent and only want to be happy and loved.

We had an enjoyable time for the two hours we were there. We noticed he had started to enjoy playing and interacting with others. I was still on guard, just in case, but I came to the realisation that his biting habit was actually brought upon by adults. Being such a cute and irresistible child, everyone was eager to interact with him. They would say 'I am coming and I am going to bite you!' So this child developed the mindset that biting was a loving response. The only way to break this was for the adults around him to stop doing it. It was also helpful to cautiously continue his exposure to other babies so that he could slowly alter the habit without too much drama or confusion.

I remember more than twenty years ago one of my dogs hated bicycles. He was not allowed to come for walks because he chased cyclists and was so strong that I could not hold him down. One day I took him to a bike track where youths practised. I tied him up very, very close to the track. He was crazy at first, but calmed down half an hour later after realising the bikes would not bother him anymore. This is the principle I thought I would apply when correcting my grandson's biting habit. When my daughter came to check on us he was more content playing on his own, going around trying every toy, and appeared not to be biting the other babies anymore. Physical punishment, such as smacking, was not necessary. This is often the case as most of children's bad habits or misdemeanours are likely learned from superior beings.

I share this story because, watching my daughter and her friends grow up, I have observed the positive effects of introducing children to spirituality. It causes them to look at life in a more meaningful way. I understand that we all try our best. My parents tried their best and I tried to find ways to raise my child to be the best person she could be. My wish for her and my son-in-law is that they become the most understanding parents to their children, and that they continue to model this positive behaviour for future generations.

My daughter still rolls her eyes in front of her friends every now and then when I invite the archangels to assist me when things get out of hand. I understand her views, as spirituality is not commonly known and is seldom practised by people her age. I know she has beliefs that need boosting. One night her car would not start after work. She was tired and desperately wanted to get home. She tried a few times but heard the sound of the battery diminishing. In her desperation, she asked Archangel Michael for help and, when she turned the key, her car started. My daughter's view is understandable. Shame still plays in her mind as this is not a common practice, but deep down in her heart she really believes in angels and inner guides. She is just being cautious as our non-believer society tends not to understand. My beliefs are not really taught in normal daily life. The mindset she exhibits shows how individuals live in fear of being criticised. But if parents were to introduce and teach children from an early age how to connect with angels and ask them for help with tasks and attaining a peaceful life, these beliefs would then become natural and the new generation would have less stress and more peace and compassion. It would create a generation of very loving children living in a wonderful peaceful world.

Acknowledgement

Extreme gratitude to Peter G. and Maryna Verbitska from the Ukraine for their professional and accomplished artistry and for their prompt response to my call for help.

Peter G.
www.classicbikenut.com

Maryna Verbitska
https://plus.google.com/103214766552484375318

My extreme gratitude to Gabie Proc, my workshop mentor, for her ongoing patience and guidance in helping me understand the importance of time duration to professionally run a workshop.

My heartfelt gratitude to Natasa for the Ultimate 48 Hour Author workshop, during which she kindly revealed her system and made book-writing fun and easy.

Natasa Denman
www.ultimate48hourauthor.com.au

www.natasadenman.com

Sources

Heal Yourself the Natural Way – Walter Last

www.amazon.com/Natural-Way-Heal-Walter-Last/dp/1571743189

Bob Doyle – Author Wealth beyond Reason

www.amazon.com/Wealth-Beyond-Reason-Bob-Doyle/dp/1412013607

Darren Linton

www.guidedbyangels.info

Kyle Gray

www.kylegray.co.uk

Don Tolman

www.amazon.com/Don-Tolman/e/B008Y26WUS

Maria Russo, Author and Founder of Forensic Healing

www.amazon.com/Natural-Way-Heal-Walter-Last/dp/1571743189

Michelle Mayur

http://www.angelwings-healing.com/about/michellemayur

Dr Sandra Cabot

www.sandracabot.com/health-books

Additional Healthy Tips – How to Lose Weight the Healthy Way

www.mayoclinic.org/healthy-lifestyle/weight-loss/in-depth/...

Bob Proctor

https://en.wikipedia.org/wiki/The_Secret_(2006_film)

Dean Jackson

www.amazon.com/Dean-Jackson/e/B00GCZDM1Q

Doreen Virtue

www.youtube.com/user/4AngelTherapy

Haim Ginott

https://en.wikipedia.org/wiki/Haim_Ginott

Wayne Dyer

www.drwaynedyer.com/wayne-dyer-quotes

Pablo Picasso

https://en.wikipedia.org/wiki/Pablo_Picasso

Self-Love

www.carolinekirk.com

https://uk.pinterest.com/explore/self-esteem

Dalai Lama

https://en.wikipedia.org/wiki/Dalai_Lama

McCarthy, Cormac (1992), All the Pretty Horses, Alfred A. Knopf, New York

Eckhart Tolle

https://en.wikipedia.org/wiki/Eckhart_Tolle

Create Healthy Boundaries

www.gypsyowlproductions.com/crown-chakra.html

Creative Inspirations

http://documents.mx/documents/the-7-chakras.html

Chakra Healing

www.mindbodygreen.com/0-91

www.reiki-for-holistic-health.com/chakra-balancing-healing.html

Angels Healing Lights

www.angeltherapy.com/blog/why-seeing-lights-sign-your-angels

Aberjhani

www.goodreads.com/.../326264-you-were-born-a-child-of-light-s-wond

www.ingramcontent.com/pod-product-compliance
Lightning Source LLC
Chambersburg PA
CBHW071529080526
44588CB00011B/1607